Living the Food-Allergic Life

T0055261

ALSO BY MARK S. FERRARA
AND FROM McFARLAND

*Barack Obama
and the Rhetoric of Hope* (2013)

Living the Food-Allergic Life

MARK S. FERRARA

Foreword by Peter F. Torrisi, M.D.

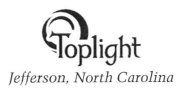

Jefferson, North Carolina

ISBN (print) 978-1-4766-9143-5
ISBN (ebook) 978-1-4766-4928-3

LIBRARY OF CONGRESS AND BRITISH LIBRARY
CATALOGUING DATA ARE AVAILABLE

Library of Congress Control Number 2023003991

Front cover images © Lightspring/OrangeVector/Shutterstock

Printed in the United States of America

Toplight is an imprint of McFarland & Company, Inc., Publishers

*Box 611, Jefferson, North Carolina 28640
www.toplightbooks.com*

For my brother Tony,
with gratitude for the deft ride up
Chippenham Parkway to the emergency room

Table of Contents

Acknowledgments

In writing this book, I am indebted to many people, among them James and Cory Ferrara, Arnaud Brichon, W. Scott Howard, Nick Boyar, Suzanne Black, Tony Ferrara, J. Jeremy Wisnewski, Wesley Graves, Paul G. Ferrara. Great thanks to readers who reviewed the manuscript in draft form: C.W. Huntington, Jr., Walter R. Coppedge, Liangmei Bao, Nicole Jones, Peter Torrisi, Cliff Edwards, Bryan Walpert, Leamor Kahanov, and Arabez Smith.

I'm appreciative of the librarians and staff members at the Cornell University Libraries in Ithaca and the Milne Library in Oneonta, New York, where this book was researched—and for the work of the editorial and production teams at Toplight Books. I remember also the young people featured in these pages who lost their lives to food allergy: Alexi Stafford, Karanbir Cheema, Sabrina Shannon, and Brooklyn Secor.

Foreword

BY PETER F. TORRISI, M.D.

Over the last three years, nothing has generated more discussion worldwide than the Covid-19 pandemic. For those gravely ill from Covid, their lungs become dysfunctional as the tiny air sacs designed to exchange oxygen flood with fluid (acute respiratory distress syndrome) and the blood pressure drops dangerously low, resulting in septic shock.

If you are wondering what this has to do with the subject of this book, both Covid and anaphylaxis involve parts of the immune system that become dysregulated, dysfunctional, or have, in other words, "gone haywire." Like our military with its multiple branches (Army, Navy, Air Force, Marines, Coast Guard), our immune system has multiple branches designed for a certain purpose that also work in concert with each other. Each part of the immune system contains a dizzying array of cells, chemicals, sometimes antibodies, and chemical messengers to carry out its task.

Our cells utilize these chemical messengers, known as cytokines, to convey information to other cells with the goal of providing the body with the necessary tools to protect, help heal injuries, and preserve the body's well-being. One can't turn on the television without being bombarded with commercials about some medicine with the final suggestion to "Ask your doctor if this is right for you." Very often, these medicines are specifically created antibodies designed to regulate and normalize our body's inappropriate and excessive number of chemical messengers which may occur in certain disease states, with the goal of reducing inflammation.

All asthmatic patients suffer from inappropriate inflammation in their airways, causing them to have difficulty breathing, and about half of those who are afflicted with asthma have some type of an allergic component. There are presently several available therapeutic antibodies that are very helpful in treating the allergic components of asthma and another medicine, Tezspire (tezepelumab-ekko), shows promise for treating those with and without an allergic component.

Almost everyone has had a bee sting at some time in their life. For those of us fortunate enough to not be allergic, we still experience localized swelling and redness—the result of the enlargement of small blood vessels in the nearby vicinity, as well as their becoming extra leaky. This response allows different cells and chemicals to escape the confines of blood vessels and do what they were designed to do—fight the invader. For people highly allergic to bee stings, the message becomes distorted and generalized. Instead of just having a local reaction, blood vessels throughout the body become dilated and leaky causing a precipitous sudden drop in blood pressure. If the swelling occurs in the throat and tongue, the airway becomes choked off leaving the person in grave danger of suffocating and dying without immediate intervention. This latter syndrome is what can occur with a very severe allergic reaction known as anaphylaxis, and, in the author's case, it occurred after accidental ingestion of the wrong food.

Having practiced as a pulmonary and critical care physician for almost forty years, I have encountered many patients who have endured anaphylaxis. It is still always very alarming to watch this occur in someone who was otherwise healthy just moments before their accidental exposure. It has been more than twenty years since I encountered the author in such a scenario, and as is often the case, I not only remember taking care of him but also the number of the bed in the ICU where he resided. In this book, the author delivers wonderful insight into the physical, social, and psychological dilemmas that people encounter living with such an illness, while also bringing hope for the future.

There has been much progress made utilizing well-controlled scientific studies which continue to increase our understanding of the biochemistry underlying different disease processes, but we clearly still have a large hill to climb before we can offer the type of medical treatment that is greatly needed in this arena.

Dr. Peter Torrisi is a pulmonary and critical care specialist in Richmond, Virginia. He graduated from the New York Medical College, completed further training at Brown University and George Washington University, and is affiliated with facilities such as Chippenham Hospital and Bon Secours St. Francis Medical Center.

Preface

There is no cure for my illness, but you won't see signs of it on my body. It leaves no scars, twists no bones, causes no quaking, yet it remains ever in the background, like a thief with a loaded gun, waiting for my guard to drop. I wish I could tell you a triumphant story, of how I overcame a deadly disease and refused to let it limit my activities, but that would be a lie. This illness looms large in my life, at every meal, but no more so than when I'm away from home. How do you make clear, to an acquaintance who invites you over for dinner or to a waiter in a foreign country, that eating a tiny amount of a forbidden food could kill you in less time than it takes to finish a meal? How do you describe what happens to the body during an allergic reaction? How do you explain that only complete avoidance of food allergens can prevent emergency medical intervention—and possibly death?

The disease that afflicts me also afflicts millions of children and adults around the world, which is why I decided to write this book, even though it forces me to confess to fear-filled thoughts that are not always rational. Although anaphylaxis may be triggered by insect stings, medicines, and even exercise, this is a story of living with anaphylaxis related to food. It is simply a true story, one that in retelling may offer little new medical insight into the disease process, but that illuminates the mind of the sufferer, and provides assurance to others struggling with eating that they are not alone. This is a story about how the body can betray you on the most basic level, in the daily need to nourish it to stay alive. This is a story of what can happen to the mind when something as elemental as hunger conjures the specter of death. This is a story needing to be told, and not because I've accomplished wonderful things in my life. I've never been nominated for a prize, won a sports championship, or built a million-dollar business. The most I've accomplished is surviving for many years in China, South Korea, and Turkey with anaphylactic food allergies, earning a doctorate in literary studies, and becoming a faculty member at a state college.

3

Living the Food-Allergic Life

Although the difficulties that I encountered finding safe meals in these and other countries—and what happened when I couldn't—are part of this story, this book is written for people striving to live healthfully with food allergies, as well as for those who care for them and want to know more about what life looks like with this invisible affliction. When anaphylaxis comes after accidentally eating the wrong food, it comes suddenly and causes the throat to close, the lungs to fill with mucus, the blood pressure to drop, consciousness to be lost, the organs to fail. Believe me, at such moments, one stares death in the eyes. Even the epinephrine auto-injectors, the plastic, spring-loaded syringes that patients thrust into the sides of their thighs in an emergency, may not provide enough relief to reverse the allergic response. I know because a jab did not save me from the ventilator in 2001.

In telling my story, I have sometimes changed the names of people to protect their privacy. The sections that recount my struggle with asthma and food allergies are, to the best of my recollection, an accurate portrayal of what I have experienced and witnessed. Yet, my story is just one among many allergic lives featured in these pages. Some of those voices belong to preteens and teenagers living with allergies to multiple foods, including common staples such as milk, eggs, wheat, and soybeans. Other voices come from parents raising children with food allergies who struggle to find daycare and schools that recognize the severity of their condition. Additional perspectives come from medical professionals, including forewordist Dr. Peter Torrisi, the cardiovascular and pulmonary disease specialist who saved my life after an accidental ingestion of tree nuts in 2001.

Although this book is not an academic study, it provides a useful overview of the allergic response in lay terms, considers causes for the rapid rise in prevalence of food allergies around the world, evaluates current treatment options, and concludes with a survey of voices reflecting on life and the transitory nature of the material world. Food allergies may develop at any stage of life, and even in their milder forms, they can be profoundly disruptive. I offer this work in the hope that it will help people living with food allergies realize that they are not alone, that their daily struggles are shared by millions of us, and that with vigilance we can live full, happy, healthy, and meaningful lives—not despite our allergies, but because of them.

CHAPTER ONE

Dancing with Anaphylaxis
-or-
The Virtues of Epinephrine

"But, by the all-powerful dispensations of providence, I have been protected beyond all human expectations or probability."
—George Washington in a 1755 letter penned after he had survived a battle in which two horses were shot from under him and four bullet holes were discovered in his coat

-◊-

One sunny spring day, an acceptance letter came from the U.S. Fulbright Commission, and in the spirit of surrender, I took a leave from graduate school to teach in Turkey, an ancient land at the crossroads of Europe and Asia. That move meant trading the big blue skies of Colorado's front range for the rugged steppes of Anatolia and the familiar patterns of life for the unknowns of Ankara, the bustling capital city in Turkey's heartland. It was the summer of 2001, and earlier that year Chief Justice William Rehnquist had sworn in George W. Bush as the forty-third American president; United Nations weapons inspectors sought (but never found) stockpiles of chemical and biological weapons in Iraq; the Taliban destroyed monumental sixth century Buddhist sculptures in the Bamiyan Valley of Afghanistan; and protests against globalization rocked the G8 summit in Genoa, Italy. Unaware that the tragedy of the September 11 terrorist attacks would soon ensnare the United States in the longest foreign wars in our country's history, Americans queued to see *Jurassic Park III* and a film about a swamp ogre named *Shrek*, tuned their television sets to new episodes of *Malcolm in the Middle* and *Buffy the Vampire Slayer*, and grooved to the beats of Destiny's Child, Alicia Keys, and Weezer.

Living the Food-Allergic Life

After packing up our one-bedroom apartment near the University of Denver in early July, my wife Savannah and I drove across the Great Plains to Virginia for what we thought would be a short visit with family while the Turkish Embassy processed our residency permits. Delays in that process meant that by mid–August, we were marooned. Shortly thereafter, an invitation arrived: Walter, beloved professor and mentor, was hosting a dinner party. Mid-to-late summers swelter in Richmond, humidity thickens the air, and the sun warms it into a steam bath. When dusk falls, the air cools and cicadas fill it with their throbbing song. On just such an evening, Walter, a debonair septuagenarian with silver hair, bright blue eyes, a short beard, and a scholarly gait, welcomed friends to his Edwardian Fan District home near Virginia Commonwealth University to share a meal and a drink or two.

In the retreating twilight heat, we gathered in his backyard garden at tables assembled off the deck. Small white candles lit the winding path leading to the back gate, and their flickering light reflected off a small pond and illuminated the statued faces of renunciates sitting in meditation under a variety of flowering trees and plants: nandina, dogwoods, pansies, hydrangeas, azaleas, camellias, and roses. Conscious of the severity of my food allergy, Walter had prepared for his guests a simple repast of baked salmon, white rice, vegetables, and a tossed salad. I understood that he had taken care to prepare a meal safe for me, but I knew that he was a vegetarian who often cooked with tree nuts, and so I chose to sip red wine and enjoy the good conversation instead. Consequently, I returned to my father's place south of the city after midnight, famished, and slightly buzzed.

Once inside, I went to the pantry, pondered shelves of canned soup, instant noodles, saltine crackers, tuna fish, jars of nuts, and cases of soft drinks, and grabbed a blue bag of mini Chips Ahoy cookies, which looked identical to the plain ones that I enjoyed at home. I still ate sweets, but only when a list of ingredients could be reviewed. On this occasion, because the packaging looked familiar, I scanned the ingredients absent-mindedly and popped a mini cookie into my mouth—and swallowed it. Almost instantly, a profound sense of impending doom swept over me. I reached for the package again, reread the label, and with darkest dismay realized that the cookies contained pecans. I rushed to the small half-bath in the hallway behind the kitchen, just a few feet from the pantry, and frantically stuck a finger down my throat in repeated, but ultimately futile, attempts to vomit them up. Knowing

6

from experience that the onset of anaphylaxis would occur within minutes, I began to murmur to myself repeatedly, "Oh, no. Oh no."

Fifteen-year-old Alexi Ryann Stafford made the same mistake, almost eighteen years later, when she ate a chewy Chips Ahoy cookie at a friend's house from a red package nearly identical to those made without peanuts, which her family had deemed "safe" for her. The fifteen-year-old from Florida with long brown hair, hazel eyes, and braces began to feel an unpleasant tingling sensation in her mouth, an early sign of an allergic reaction to food. She went home immediately where her condition deteriorated rapidly. As she struggled for breath, her frightened mother, Kellie Travers-Stafford, called for an ambulance and injected Alexi with two shots of epinephrine. While waiting for the paramedics to arrive, "for what felt like an eternity," Alexi slipped into anaphylactic shock, lost consciousness, and stopped breathing. Within ninety minutes of eating a single peanut butter cookie, she was dead.

Devastated, her mother, who had dedicated herself to keeping Alexi away from peanuts, took to social media to "spread awareness so that this horrible mistake doesn't happen again."[1] "As a mother," she wrote, "who diligently taught her the ropes of what was okay to ingest and what was not, I feel lost and angry because she knew her limits and was aware of familiar packaging, she knew what 'safe' was."[2] Alexi's mother shared two pictures, one showing the Reese's variety that killed her daughter and another showing the regular chewy kind—and they had strikingly similar packaging. The company had failed, Travers-Stafford asserted, to clearly warn of the presence of ingredients potentially fatal to many people: "A small added indication on the pulled back flap on a familiar red package wasn't enough to call out to her that there was 'peanut product' in the cookies before it was too late."[3]

I was older than Alexi and had survived three previous anaphylactic reactions, so it never occurred to me to call an ambulance and wait for it to reach my father's home in the remote suburbs of Chesterfield County. Instead, after two to three minutes of trying unsuccessfully to induce a gag reflex to purge my stomach of the allergen and spare the body the worst of the reaction to come, I began to panic as the specter of past exposures arose in my mind: the sudden inability to breathe as lungs fill with mucus, the swelling shut of the throat and other air pathways, and the disorientation and confusion that clouds consciousness as blood pressure drops and cells and organs are deprived of oxygen.

Less than five minutes had elapsed before I hastily explained to Savannah, now in blue cotton pajamas and ready for bed, that I needed to get to a hospital emergency room as quickly as possible. I knew it normally took about thirty minutes to reach the hospital on the winding roads leading out of my father's neighborhood, and by that time the onset of anaphylaxis would make me a danger to myself and others behind the wheel. Having grown up in China, a country with many alternate options for transportation (bicycles, scooters, buses, taxis, trains, airplanes), Savannah had not yet learned to drive. Even if she had, it would have been in a vehicle with an automatic transmission, and our base model Honda Civic had a four-speed manual gearbox.

Had he not been out of town for a conference, I would have awoken my father and gotten him to speed me to Chippenham Medical Center in his sports car. With precious time slipping away, I shook my younger brother Tony awake instead. "I've accidently eaten pecans," I explained with fevered urgency, "you have to get me to the hospital." Still in the fog of deep sleep, Tony rose from the beige couch in the living room where he had crashed in front of the television and began to search for his car keys and shoes. We quickly contemplated a run to a nearby private urgent care facility that was closer than the hospital, but fortunately I was still thinking clearly enough to know that an outpatient medical center might not be open at that time of night, and in any case, it would probably not be equipped to handle anaphylaxis. Before Tony could find both shoes, I hurried him out of the house toward our car and urged Savannah to join us knowing that any further delay would reduce chances of survival.

Behind the wheel with one shoe on, his long sandy brown hair disheveled, Tony raced out of the driveway and flew down the backroads. I held the blue vinyl handrail on the a-pillar with my right hand—and clutched a black medicine bag containing two epinephrine auto-injectors in the other. Concerned that Tony's aggressive driving on winding backroads might get us wrapped around a tree, I asked him to slow down a bit. But when we reached Beach Road and turned onto Route 10, a main thoroughfare, I was finding it harder to breathe. I grabbed an EpiPen, slid it out of the clear plastic case, and removed the yellow safety cap. Tony pushed the underpowered Civic down the highway, and we zoomed by streetlights that grew brighter, then dimmer, as we passed underneath them.

Halfway to the hospital, I started having to really pull for air. Without hesitation, I loosened the belt, dropped the tan slacks to my knees, and thrust the EpiPen into the side of my scrawny thigh. Click! The sudden, forceful jab of the needle surprised me, but I held the injector firmly in place for several seconds as required. After slowly pulling the needle out, I felt no relief, and soon my breathing grew more labored. When we had lived in Shanghai, I explained my food allergy to Savannah, but she had never seen an allergic reaction to food. As my throat and tongue swelled, and confused disorientation set in, I began to wonder if she would be made a young widow in the United States before we could make it to Turkey.

Ignoring traffic rules and speed limits in the middle of the night, Tony got us to the hospital in record time. A police car had tailed the speeding Honda up Chippenham Highway, but perhaps sensing a medical emergency, the officer did not pull us over. As Tony entered the traffic circle at the emergency room entrance, I was already in shock. Holding up my britches with the right hand (because it never occurred to me to button and zip them up), I have a hazy recollection of running through the sliding glass doors that opened automatically into the emergency waiting area. Glancing to my right, I locked eyes for a moment with a patient in the waiting room. He expressed no anger as I darted for the double doors leading toward the treatment rooms, thus bypassing registration and triage at the front desk. Rather, his concerned alarm suggested that I was in serious trouble. I had no way to know it, but I had already turned blue from a lack of oxygen.

Falling to my knees, I struck the treatment room doors with my left fist to be let in. As they opened, an attendant emergency room physician arrived and asked me what had happened. Instead of telling her that I was having an anaphylactic reaction to pecans (the obvious thing to say), I confessed to smoking cannabis earlier in the evening, which while true was quite unrelated to the emergency at hand. It's hard to explain, but in the fog of shock, I was overcome with an irrational fear that the copious drugs soon to be administered to treat anaphylaxis—epinephrine, antihistamines, cortisone, albuterol, and other medications— would have negative synergistic effects with that herb! That misdirected worry, and the expression on the attendant physician's face at the mention of cannabis (which I recollect as a look of "well, you clearly deserve what's happening to you") was the last thing I remember, before everything went black.

-◊-

Living the Food-Allergic Life

More than fifty million people in the United States suffer from allergies of some kind, from the unpleasant symptoms of hay fever and eczema to chronic asthma and anaphylaxis.[4] Allergies occur when the immune system overresponds to environmental substances normally harmless to most people (dust mites, pollen, mold, animal dander, insect venom, latex, food, and medicine). Allergens that elicit immune responses in the skin result in dermatitis, and they cause sneezing and congestion when they enter the nose and throat. Food antigens that enter the digestive tract cause abdominal cramps, nausea, intestinal inflammation, vomiting, and diarrhea. When environmental allergens reach the trachea, bronchi, and lungs, they trigger wheezing, broncho-constriction, and asthma.[5]

The first time the body encounters an allergen, normally little or no reaction occurs. The immune system, however, generates antibod-ies (*called immunoglobin E or IgE*) that are stored in tissue and blood cells. When that allergen is encountered again, those antibodies pounce on it and release powerful inflammatory chemicals such as histamine that move throughout the body and cause allergic symptoms ranging from mild hives, itchiness, nasal congestion, and watery eyes to swelling of the throat and airways, allergic asthma, and anaphylaxis.[6] With the onset of prolonged immune activation, hours and sometimes days after the introduction of an antigen, mast and neighboring cells can settle on tissue surfaces where they secrete chemicals that sustain inflammation and damage tissue.

Although no longer the debilitating disease that it was before the advent of albuterol inhalers in 1981, asthma still causes more than half a million hospitalizations per year in the United States alone.[7] Asthma and food allergies often coexist, and although quality data remains elusive, many countries have reported significant increases in the prevalence of food allergies over the last few decades, with some estimates suggesting that they affect 10 percent of adults and 8 percent of children in some parts of the world today.[8] Growing public awareness of food allergies has produced many positive advancements, such as nut-free classrooms and the removal of peanuts and tree nuts from airliners, but many people do not fully appreciate the ways in which anaphylactic allergies impact physical and mental well-being.

When food, medication, insect stings, or exercise trigger anaphylaxis, mast and neighboring cells circulate through the whole body and cause allergic manifestations far from the site of entry. Life-threatening symptoms often appear within minutes of exposure, as the immune system releases a flood of chemicals that lead to anaphylactic shock. During anaphylaxis, the allergic individual may experience itchy rashes, obstructive swelling of the tongue, drooling, difficulty breathing, throat tightening, uterine contractions, and a sense of impending doom. As reduced blood circulation deprives the body of oxygen and nutrients, blood pressure falls, the skin turns pale or blue, the pulse becomes difficult to detect, and the patient experiences nausea and vomiting, along with confusion, dizziness, and even fainting (a great mercy, in my experience, for anyone in such dire straits). Without prompt medical attention, death can occur shortly after the onset of symptoms due to the rapid inflammation of bronchial tubes, the closure of breathing passages, and the swelling of the vocal cords that close off the trachea. The only way for severely allergic people to prevent anaphylaxis is to practice *total avoidance of even trace amounts of food allergens.*[9]

The drug of choice for treating anaphylaxis is epinephrine, but the longer one delays treatment with it, the more likely anaphylaxis is to prove fatal. Waiting to use the drug makes it less effective, because as blood circulation slows, so does the delivery of epinephrine.[10] Surviving systemic anaphylaxis requires prompt emergency care in a facility with trained physicians and equipment for intubation (insertion of a tube through the mouth and into the airway so that patients may be placed on a ventilator to assist with breathing). The Covid-19 pandemic has raised awareness about the lifesaving potential of ventilators, but as cases peaked and hospitals filled in 2020 and 2021, people with food-induced anaphylaxis found themselves in competition for these resources in emergency situations. Even after allergic symptoms abate following prompt treatment, a second allergic wave occurs in up to 28 percent of anaphylactic reactions.[11] In rare cases, anaphylactic rebounds may continue over several days. Having a history of reactions to trace amounts of food antigens, experiencing reactions away from home, being a teenager or young adult, and having allergies to peanuts, tree nuts, shellfish, fish, and milk—these factors increase the risk of fatal food-induced anaphylaxis.

-◊-

During the momentous year of 1969 into which I was born, the American counterculture expanded into mainstream society, hippie communes and "back-to-the-land" intentional communities sprang up across the nation, enraged Vietnam protestors demonstrated against the first draft lottery since World War II, and the Woodstock Music

Festival brought youthful experimentations with free love and psychedelics into popular culture. That year, the Apollo 11 spaceship landed two astronauts on the moon, the Mariner 6 and 7 probes reconnoitered the surface of Mars, Willie Mays hit his 600th career home run, and John Lennon and Yoko Ono held a "Bed-In" for peace in Amsterdam as the Cold War grew even chillier after a Soviet submarine collided with the USS *Gato* in the Barents Sea. I have a particular fondness for 1969, because it was the only year of my life relatively free from asthma and allergies.

By this time, decades of synthetic pesticide use from the 1940s onward had contaminated water, soil, and vegetation and had proved toxic to birds, fish, insects, and other organisms. In the early 1970s, the Environmental Protection Agency banned the insecticide DDT—regarded today as a probable carcinogen—due to its tendency to accumulate in fatty tissues, its ability to travel long distances in the upper atmosphere, and its persistence in the environment. Before the passage of the Clean Water Act of 1972, only about one third of American waterways remained safe for swimming and fishing.[12] Pollution from vehicles and the combustion of fossil fuels created smog in urban areas such as Los Angeles and New York City, and burning leaded gasoline exposed tens of millions of young children to a variety of toxins, including tetraethyl lead, a highly toxic compound linked to complications later in life including lower IQ, learning disabilities, hyperactivity, and behavioral problems.[13]

By the close of the 1970s, the Environmental Protection Agency had banned synthetic PCBs used as coolants and lubricants in a variety of products (electrical appliances, fluorescent lighting ballasts, transformers and capacitors, caulking compounds, cable insulation, paint) because they caused immunological and neurobehavioral changes in children and cancer in animals. Many of those products manufactured before 1979 remain in use today.[14] The Love Canal neighborhood in Niagara Falls, New York, built atop a toxic waste dump, exposed unsuspecting residents to contaminants through vapors emanating from basements. Meanwhile, the meltdown of a reactor at the Three Mile Island nuclear power plant outside of Harrisburg, Pennsylvania, alerted the American public to the dangers of radiation-induced illnesses, which threatened those living in the vicinity of such power stations, and it highlighted the challenges of cleaning up nuclear accidents.

The prevalence of childhood asthma and allergies dramatically increased during the 1960s and 1970s, an unfortunate fact attributable to exposure to ozone, diesel exhaust, and tobacco smoke; to a rise in the frequency of viral respiratory infections; to obesity and lack of exercise; to decreased contact with microorganisms during early life (the so-called "hygiene hypothesis").[15] But environmental pollution wasn't the only thing making children and adults sick. The large-scale production of processed foods required high heat and synthetic additives, and they changed the way our meals looked, tasted, and smelled.

Artificial coloring, preservatives, stabilizers, emulsifiers, solvents, anticaking agents, artificial sweeteners, and other additives are correlated with higher rates of cancer and other health problems (including obesity, heart disease, dental cavities, Type 2 diabetes, and organ damage).[16] Readers of a certain age will remember—in addition to corduroy bell-bottoms, tight-fitting patterned polyester shirts, and Pinto automobiles—Swanson TV dinners, Cheez Whiz, Wonder Bread, Fruit Loops cereal, Carnation Breakfast Bars, Hunt's Manwich sauce, Jeno's Pizza Rolls, Shake 'n Bake coating mix, and other processed foods that quickly became part of the American dietary landscape.

-◊-

In 1969, my father's family lived in Syracuse, New York. Residents of the Village of Syracuse and the town of Salina incorporated as the City of Syracuse in 1847, nearly two centuries after the Jesuit priest Simon Le Moyne discovered salt springs near Onondaga Lake in 1654 on a site first occupied by Native Americans (the Haudenosaunee) who grew corn, beans, and squash and lived in long semi-permanent communal houses. When commercial salt production in the area accelerated following the opening of the Erie Canal in 1825, Syracuse became known as "Salt City." During the mid-to-late nineteenth century, the city was also an epicenter of the abolitionist movement and an important waypoint along the Underground Railroad.

When the Erie Canal, which once ran through the center of town, ceased to be a viable transportation route in the early-to-mid twentieth century, this once prosperous upstate urban center fell into decline. Industries built around salt production, agriculture, typewriter manufacturing, and automobile-making relocated their headquarters and production facilities to states with lower tax rates. Syracuse, along with much of the Great Lakes region, suffered rapid population loss and deindustrialization during the late 1970s and early 1980s and became part of the "Rust Belt." The geographical proximity of Syracuse to the Great Lakes meant that residents enjoyed only 160 sunny days per year, and long winters filled with lake-effect snow made the city drab and dreary for months at a time. Like many descendants of ethnic immigrants in the post–World War II era, my mother and father, both from Italian-American families, grew up trying to fit in with mainstream American culture, rather than preserving the language and traditions of their European homelands. Their parents expected them to work hard; to avail themselves of educational opportunities provided by local community colleges, colleges, and universities; and to enter the expanding middle class.

One of five siblings, my father attended a private Catholic preparatory school, gained admission to Le Moyne College, and went on to earn a doctorate in organic chemistry at Syracuse University. Later in life, he found some renown as the director of Virginia's forensic laboratories, which became the first capable of using DNA fingerprinting to solve crimes by creating database profiles that could be matched to previously convicted sex offenders. His role in innovating that technology is highlighted in the made-for-television film *A Life Interrupted: The Debbie Smith Story* (2007). A man of medium height and build with dark hair, thick glasses, a long nose, and a penchant for women and fast cars, he met my mother at Le Moyne College, they married, and remained that way for about eight years. My father liked to joke that I was a rough looking newborn: face bruised from the trauma of birth, chubby going on plump, with a head of matted brown-black hair that rose from the eyebrows and reached to the back of my neck. (In middle age, that mane has retreated to a narrow ring around the back and sides of my head!)

My mother, a petite five-foot-three Mediterranean beauty with an olive complexion, brown eyes, and long dark hair worn straight (like Cher when she sang with Sonny), graduated from college, worked as a registered nurse, earned a master's degree in psychiatric nursing from the University of Virginia, and became a teacher and program administrator. She came from a dysfunctional family rife with alcoholism and mental illness, which in many ways was the opposite of the staid, nurturing, and conservative home of my father. Part of the allure of my father to my mother would have been the open-heartedness of his parents, who always treated her as their daughter. Decades after my parents' divorce, Mom retained a special place in their affections that my stepmother could never quite eclipse (though she stole my father's heart). The repercussions of my mother and father's divorce echoed throughout my childhood and still resonate today, ten years after the loss of my Dad to brain cancer.

14

Chapter One. Dancing with Anaphylaxis

Mom enjoys recounting the story of going into labor with me during a late February snowstorm. Just a few months from completing his dissertation, Dad rushed her to the hospital, deposited her into an empty wheelchair at the entrance, and pushed her through the corridor to admissions. He eagerly turned over the whole messy affair of birth to the doctors and nurses. That episode, to my mother's mind, tacitly brings to the fore my father's absenteeism during much of my early life. In the late 1960s, men seldom witnessed the birth of their children, and I like to imagine Pop entering a smoke-filled waiting room full of anxious fathers-to-be, his hair parted to the side, a cigarette clutched between his fingers, and a bouncing knee that betrayed a constantly churning mind. Although I appeared a healthy child, illness struck before my first birthday and a diagnosis of childhood asthma swiftly followed.

-◊-

The most common triggers for asthma include tobacco smoke, dust mites, pet dander, pollens and molds, chemical irritants in the workplace, and air pollution. Once sensitized to an environmental allergen, repeated exposure to it can lead to chronic airway constriction and inflammation that produces wheezing, breathlessness, and coughing, especially at night and in the early morning. Without proper medical care, long-term exposure to allergens can cause permanent damage to lung tissue, reduction in lung function, severe breathing discomfort, and lower resistance to infection. Cold air, physical exercise, and the arousal of strong emotions, such as anger or fear, may also precipitate the onset of symptoms. Asthma can be mild, interfere with daily activities, or become life-threatening. During an asthma attack, the restricted passage of air into the lungs results in shortness of breath that may last from a few minutes to several days. Severe attacks close off airways completely and are potentially fatal. The World Health Organization estimates that 262 million people around the world suffered from asthma in 2019, and children, ethnic minorities, and the urban poor have the highest probability of developing it. Asthma still claims the lives of more than 450,000 people every year.[17]

Allergic diseases run in families and strong genetic correlations bind asthma and food allergies together. When both parents have asthma, their children are more likely to develop it. The more types of allergies found in families, and the greater number of members affected, the more probable that other relatives will also have them. Having a sibling with allergies gives a child about a 15 percent risk of developing them. If one parent has them, that figure rises to 30 to 50 percent, and to 60 to 80 percent when both do.[18] Although children may outgrow some allergies, including those to foods such as milk and eggs, otherwise healthy people may develop food allergies in adulthood, which usually means they will persist for life and most often involve nuts, seafood, fruits (banana, kiwi, mango, peach, pineapple, strawberry), or vegetables (eggplant, avocado, celery, cucumber, garlic, beetroot, cabbage, carrot, mushroom, onion, peppers).

Although anyone may develop food allergies that result in anaphylaxis at any time during their lives, those with a family or a personal history of allergic diseases are at greatest risk. My father and mother suffered from environmental allergies most of their adult lives— whereas my childhood asthma was followed by the onset of extreme food allergies in adolescence. Children with both of these conditions are more likely to have near-fatal or fatal reactions to food, in part due to the difficulty of managing food allergies at a young age and because their asthma is more likely to be severe.[19] Food allergies also occur more frequently in individuals with relatives who suffer from allergic diseases such as eczema, hay fever, and asthma or who have pre-existing allergies to food, insect venom, latex, and other allergens.

During the late 1960s and early 1970s, medical professionals were often skeptical of diagnoses of food allergies and commonly regarded patient claims of having them as a symptom of hypochondria or anxiety disorder. Research scientists therefore conducted little research on food allergies, and the unreliability of skin testing and food-specific serum IgE values made them poor diagnostic tools (due to their weak correlation with oral food-challenge outcomes).[20] These and other attitudes thwarted investigation into the causes, symptoms, and possible treatments for a wide range of food allergies that suddenly began to appear in children. Although this relative lack of concern about food allergies may seem irresponsible, they affected only about 1 percent of the population in the 1970s. Schools did not make special accommodations for food-allergic students, allergen warnings did not exist on food labels, and restaurant staff had scant experience serving customers who could die before finishing a meal.

Starting in the early 1980s, a rapid rise in mild to potentially deadly food allergies, along with rates of asthma, led some medical professionals to regard them as part of a "second wave of the allergy epidemic."[21] Food-related allergic reactions now constitute the single leading cause of anaphylaxis treated in American emergency rooms.[22] Pollution, sanitized living environments, obesity, processed food and food additives, and vitamin and nutrient deficiencies have contributed to that epidemic. Effective and widely available treatments for severe food allergies remain almost as distant a prospect as a cure, but much has changed for the better. Few trained medical personnel today would respond with disbelief about food allergy, and the correlation between asthma and food allergy is much better understood.

According to the "hygiene hypothesis," food allergies stem from misdirected immune responses by parts of the body ready to fight germs and parasites.[23] Our uber-clean modern lifestyles, the theory goes, have deprived our immune systems of the necessity of fighting parasitic infestation. Instead, the body targets innocent proteins, resulting in allergies. Vaccinations, antibiotics, cleansers, sanitized living spaces, the movement from farms (where children played and worked in the dirt and lived among domesticated animals) to urban landscapes of concrete and steel are thought to have contributed to increasing rates of allergy in post-industrial societies. The fact that we've protected ourselves from parasite infections may mean we've compromised immune systems adapted to manage the consequences of hosting parasitic worms during most of our evolutionary history. Advocates of this hypothesis often draw support from the fact that the prevalence of food allergy rises as countries develop to post-industrial levels. Differences in food allergy prevalence also occur within countries; in urban areas of China, for instance, people have more allergies than in rural ones.[24]

Support for the hygiene hypothesis comes from studies showing that hookworms can cure or alleviate allergies and allergic diseases, including inflammatory bowel disorders, asthma, and food allergy.[25] Parasitic worms produce saliva that seems to change the immune system and stop the body from overreacting to triggers that cause allergies. To test the association between intestinal parasites and food allergies and intolerances, Dr. James Logan at the London School of Hygiene and Tropical Medicine infected himself with hookworms. Logan, who suffered from a food intolerance that prevented him from eating bread without becoming ill, found that afterward he could tolerate pizza and breadsticks without nauseating side effects.[26] The idea of "parasite therapy" to treat food allergies may sound crazy or just plain gross, but I'd take it (or should I say "them"), if it meant accidently ingesting a small quantity of tree nuts would not trigger anaphylaxis. Readers, of course, should not infect themselves or others with parasites to test this hypothesis.

-◊-

17

Living the Food-Allergic Life

It is extremely difficult, perhaps impossible, to prevent severe food allergies from negatively impacting quality of life, but one grace of food-induced anaphylaxis is the possibility of remaining virtually symptom free (unlike with other chronic illnesses such as COPD, diabetes, cystic fibrosis, dementia), so long as the food antigens that trigger immune response are absolutely avoided. The "invisible" nature of the disease presents its own challenges, but the courageous act of facing death with every meal can propel one to discover deeper meaning in life. With prompt medical attention, one can survive anaphylaxis, as I have on several occasions, though it may mean enduring intubation to keep oxygen flowing throughout the body by forcing air into the lungs. On the other hand, the terrifying nature of anaphylaxis leaves lingering psychological aftereffects ranging from eating disorders rooted in severe anxiety to post-traumatic stress disorder, which develops in some people after shocking, frightening, and dangerous events. The fact that 75 percent of people living with severe food allergies assert that they would benefit from mental health counseling speaks to the difficulty of successfully managing this condition.[27] It also points to the need to better address the repercussions of surviving anaphylaxis and the struggle to return to some measure of normalcy in its wake.

The autobiographical accounts that follow are reconstructed from the memory of illness, and for me they constitute unpleasant forays into the past that evoke mostly forgotten periods of physical suffering: the asthmatic child wheezily gasping for breath for hours and sometimes days; sterile, cold hospital rooms; oxygen tents, IV drips, nebulizer treatments, repeated injections, beeping machinery; and the boney, four-eyed asthmatic kid chosen last for team activities in gym class. With each remembrance, we reconstruct events out of lingering traces in the mind. Unlike computers that store data for later retrieval, human memories "fade-to-gist" over time, and the details of our experiences quickly wane, though our basic understanding of them persists longer. Memory also borrows from imagination and generates details to build a picture of past events, as in the case of false confessions of a crime later exonerated by evidence or in mistaken eyewitness testimonies during criminal trials.

Neurons begin to grow in the frontal lobe at around eight or nine months of age, though children rarely form memories based on experiences before the age of two or three. As a result, memories of early childhood straddle the actual and the imagined, and they often constitute reenactments of events supplemented by the recollections of friends and family members, which grow fainter and more dreamlike with each passing year.[28] Despite these limitations, the vignettes that follow highlight the struggle of many children, teens, and adults with asthma and food allergies. Given that true events are warped and woven through the prism of memory and time, to bolster those accounts and to improve their fidelity, I have augmented personal recollections with family photos, personal diaries, family stories, and academic research. In other words, in writing this book, I'm "Diving into the Wreck" of memory. I have read the book of myths, loaded the camera, and I "go down / Rung after rung" to probe the depths of remembrance and discover what poet Adrienne Rich called "the wreck and not the story of the wreck / the thing itself and not the myth."[29]

-◊-

At the time of my first asthma attack, we lived in graduate student housing at Syracuse University. Allergens in our apartment did not trigger that attack. It happened in my grandparents' home at the edge of Onondaga Park. The drainage issues that encouraged the growth of mold and mildew in the basement, combined with the antique furnishings and musty rugs that my grandparents (local upholsterers) kept, prompted the asthma attack that led to my first hospitalization at nine months of age. Whatever the trigger, during an extended visit to my grandparents' home in late 1969 (designed to give my father time alone to complete his dissertation), Mom and I slept in the spare bedroom. One night, I awoke with intense shortness of breath (dyspnea) and tightening of the chest, which gave the appearance of suffocation. Those symptoms became so pronounced that my mother and grandparents rushed me to the pediatric emergency room at Upstate Medical Center—now part of the State University of New York system for which I teach. Mom remembers the terror of being a new mother helplessly watching a child gasp for breath. She feared for my life when the nebulizers and steroids available at the time did little to reverse the allergic response.

Since I was less than a year old, my pediatrician, Dr. Levy, did not want to draw arterial blood gases from my tiny wrist. Over the next two decades, though, I would endure that painful procedure on many occasions. It required the insertion of a long, thin needle into the radial artery to get an accurate measurement of oxygen and carbon dioxide in the blood. If the technician missed the artery the first time, the needle had to be withdrawn and reinserted as often as necessary to get a pulsatile of dark red blood. As ill as I was at that time, Mom remembers me reaching a hand out between the bars of the crib to comfort a much sicker child with a brain tumor. It has been my curious experience many times since then that, when hospitalized, I've frequently been overcome with compassion for the suffering of others. (The last time I remember such a feeling was in 1997 after getting food poisoning in South Korea. A local family had brought their *halmoni*, grandmother, to that crowded emergency room in Masan, and immediately a tremendous sympathy arose for her in my heart. When he came back to check on me, I asked the doctor how she was doing. "She's probably not going to make it," replied Dr. Kim with sadness in his voice.)

Because I was so sick, Mom tearfully pleaded with Dr. Levy, a man in his mid-forties with dark hair, brown eyes, and a reputation as an empathetic physician, to find a way to help me. "I'm doing the best I can, Nikki," he replied, "but I can't guarantee he will live." In my mother's recounting of this episode, she turned to prayer: "Lord, if you cannot spare this child, you had better take me with him; there's no way I'll endure his death." After repeated injections of epinephrine halted that attack, I was released from the hospital three to four days later. Dr. Levy's verdict: bronchiolitis (a pre-asthma diagnosis) thought to be allergic in nature. "It's a good thing you came in when you did, Nikki," he said, relieved. Timely intervention, I would discover in later years, often meant the difference between life and death.

-◊-

My father graduated a few months later and took a position as a research chemist with DuPont in Waynesboro, Virginia. From then on, we visited upstate New York one or two times a year. Located 450 miles south of Syracuse, Waynesboro lies in the heart of the Shenandoah Valley. Native Americans (Piedmont Siouans, Catawbas, Shawnee, Delaware, Cherokees, Susquehannocks) had settled there long before the arrival of Europeans. Lured by its excellent farmland, German and Scots-Irish settlers fenced off the valley during the eighteenth century and established trade centers linked to the Pennsylvania Germans, who had preceded them. In a futile attempt to retain their territory, Native Americans launched attacks on settler farmsteads until the start of the American Revolution, but thereafter official records note no indigenous people living in the area. During the Civil War, General Stonewall Jackson fought off Union troops near Waynesboro, though two years later General Sheridan delivered a series of stinging defeats to Confederate troops in 1864 and wrested the valley from them, victories which contributed to the reelection of Abraham Lincoln in November.[30]

In that rustic locale, near the Blue Ridge Parkway, Skyline Drive, Appalachian Trail, and Shenandoah National Park, the DuPont chemical company built a large plant (now owned by Koch Industries) on the eastern shore of the South River. In that facility, DuPont developed and manufactured polymers, synthetic rubbers, and synthetic fibers (Orlon Lycra, Nomex, Vespel, Permasep, and Nylon). From 1929 to 1950, storm sewers washed mercury used in the manufacturing process from the soil, along with groundwater surrounding the site, into the South River and the Shenandoah River. A $50 million settlement in 2017, in which DuPont admitted no fault, was used to improve water quality, protect the land, and enhance recreational opportunities such as fishing.[31] Our years in Waynesboro were generally healthy ones for me. The climate is sunnier and more temperate than Syracuse, and Mom liked the small ranch-style home with a brick façade they purchased there, even though her family in Utica teasingly referred to Waynesboro as "the boondocks."

Photographs show a brown-skinned boy on his second birthday with a bowl haircut in a sailor pullover, tied with a red ribbon around the collar, cutting a slice of chocolate cake. Behind the boy, carefully guiding the knife in his hand, his mother, attired in a candy-cane dress accented with a red, white, and blue cloth belt, her hair straight, parted down the middle, cut just past the shoulder. The white walls of the kitchen are empty, the wooden cabinets closed. A yellow and white linoleum tablecloth covers the kitchen table. The cake has a single large white candle, more like those found in candleholders on a formal dinner table than the smaller, colored ones used for birthday cakes. In another photo, the boy's large brown eyes, slightly almond-shaped, droop at the outside; his uneven front bangs suggest a home haircut by an untutored hand. In front of the white mantle, a large black vase filled with ornate dried grasses. The boy's fingers move toward a rubber pacifier with a ring the color of fossil-filled amber. He wears a white shirt with long sleeves and no collar, and his baby overalls have a clear plastic button on each strap and a blue-green zipper down the middle. Perhaps due to the clean mountain air, or because my parents had bought a newer home, I had no allergic reactions in Waynesboro that required hospitalization.

Mom does recall once making a peanut butter sandwich for lunch and finding me vomiting on the stairs later. It's unclear if this episode was an early indication of the food allergy that developed in adolescence, for I once tolerated peanuts and peanut butter. Recent blood tests, however, returned a Class 2 positive response to peanuts (compared to Class 3 positive for pecan and macadamia; Class 4 strongly positive for walnut, Brazil nut, coconut, and cashew; and Class 5 strongly positive for almond and hazelnut). Unfortunately, no test can predict the type or severity of a reaction to food allergens based solely on class numbers. Out of an abundance of caution, I removed peanuts from my diet after last enduring anaphylaxis. That said, I still feed peanuts to chipmunks around the small pagoda where I write during the summer, and occasionally enjoy a Chick-fil-a sandwich cooked in refined peanut oil without incident. *Refined* peanut oil is generally considered safe for most peanut allergic persons, since the protein trigger is removed during the extraction process (unlike in *unrefined* peanut oils that are cold-pressed, expressed, expelled, and extruded from peanut—and pose a real danger to those with peanut allergy).[32] One whiff of an opened snack jar of mixed nuts or tree nuts being cooked, by contrast, fills me with foreboding.

-◊-

After the elimination of my father's position, along with many others at DuPont, we moved from the seclusion of Waynesboro to a small townhome in sprawling Centreville about 25 miles southwest of downtown Washington, D.C. In that older row home, the environmental allergies returned and drew me into a cycle of yearly hospitalizations that would continue until adolescence when the advent of albuterol inhalers kept those allergic responses from spiraling into severe attacks. At certain times during the year, particularly in the spring and fall, my nose became so congested that I could force air through it only with great effort and a good deal of unpleasant noise. My breath often reeked because of that congestion, like that of someone with a terrible cold. Following allergists' guidelines, Mom, a germ-conscious nurse, dust-proofed my bedroom and put terrycloth over the air vents, but most of my memories of illness from those days are of the cold and hollow steel safety bars of hospital beds, IV drips taped to a boarded arm, the smell of hospital cleaning supplies, and sponge baths by attentive nurses in white uniforms. Most vivid of all, the slow onset of asthma attacks that worsened with the wheezing, dehydration, and vomiting of forced fluids, which led to hospital admission and a week's long recovery process. My body still carries the invisible marks of childhood asthma and allergies and the loss of appetite that went with them: stunted growth, remarkable thinness (125 pounds at 5'7"), slight barrel-chestedness, diminished lung capacity, acne-prone skin, a susceptibility to infection (particularly of the sinuses), and daily bouts of repetitive sneezing.

The drugs commonly used to treat asthma in the 1970s and early 1980s caused mood swings, drowsiness, depression, and anxiety in many patients, in addition to other side effects. Doctors often prescribed Prednisone to treat the swelling associated with dangerous allergic responses, but it could cause nausea, headaches, acne, irregular heartbeat, bloody stools, and muscle cramps.[33] Theophylline pills and Marax liquid (which contained ephedra) helped to manage the symptoms of asthma, but they could result in seizures, blurred vision, chest pains, persistent vomiting, high blood pressure, and difficulty urinating.[34] The Dimetapp cough suppressant might have tasted like candied grapes, but it could generate restlessness, memory problems, and loss of appetite, while the Benadryl that alleviated itchiness and running eyes and noses caused fatigue and constipation.[35]

Primatene Mist, an over-the-counter inhaler, provided only the scantest relief during an asthma attack by treating the symptoms (not the underlying condition), thereby permitting repeated attacks that could permanently damage lung tissue. The side effects of Primatene Mist included headache, nervousness, vomiting, dizziness, and in rare cases sudden worsening of breathing problems or asthma (paradoxical bronchospasm). In 2011, after fifty years of availability, Primatene Mist, which contains epinephrine, was removed from drugstore shelves due to its ozone-depleting propellant, though it was reintroduced in 2019.[36] None of the national guidelines on asthma treatment recommend inhaled epinephrine and using it too frequently may overstimulate the heart. Newer medicines better manage allergic asthma and help to prevent hospitalization, but asthma-related deaths still occur with considerable frequency, especially in low- and lower-middle income countries where those medications may not be available or affordable.

-◊-

Whereas I have only vague recollections of Waynesboro, among them sinkholes in the backyard surrounding a metal swing set painted in bright colors, my memory becomes fixed and focused in Centreville, a sprawling suburb of the nation's capital filled with townhouses, condos, and industrial buildings. The frenetic pace of life, interminable traffic lights, and seemingly limitless number of shopping centers and corporate franchises (from restaurants to clothing stores) make the city difficult to tolerate for long. Out of this suburban wasteland, one can barely conjure the tiny farming village with a general store and a tavern that the Virginia General Assembly chartered as a town in 1792. The *Washington Star* described Centreville in 1914 as a "stagnant and drowsy" village still bearing wounds (bullet-pitted walls and shot-riven trees) and scars (sunken graves) from the War Between the States.[37] The advent of the automobile turned Centreville into a site for country homes within reach of a major metropolitan area, and by the mid-to-late 1930s, suburbanization meant that subdivisions of catalog kit homes had popped up along Lee Highway.

We moved to Centreville after Dad took a position as a bench chemist for the newly created state Division of Consolidated Laboratory Services, which included the Bureau of Forensic Science. Over decades, he rose through the ranks to become director of an expanded Department of Forensic Science that provided laboratory services to over 400 law enforcement agencies in the Commonwealth. In his honor, the central laboratory facility in Richmond was renamed the Paul B. Ferrara Building in 2011.[38] At this time, though, his career in public safety was just beginning. My mother, who had worked as a public health nurse in Waynesboro, found fulltime employment as a community health nurse in nearby Warrenton and managed to raise two children (after the birth of my brother Paul in late 1970) with limited assistance from my father. To make health calls in rural Fauquier County, she drove an army green Volkswagen station wagon that we affectionately called "old Nellie."

On my first day of school, shortly before my mother and father divorced, a teacher mistakenly put me on the wrong bus home. When the bus emptied, the driver simply let me off with the last student passengers. I recall standing on a busy street corner, which I did not recognize, being scared, and starting to cry. Evidently, I peed myself before a kind woman rescued me. When she first approached, I recited the lesson that every young child learns: "My mother told me never to talk to strangers."

The split-level townhouse my parents had purchased in Centreville featured a modular symmetrical design befitting the burgeoning burbs. As you walked through the front door of the second unit near the end of the row, a steep staircase led up to the bedrooms and to a small bathroom. To the right, you saw a modest first floor living area with a sofa and a television. A sliding glass door opened onto a long, narrow patch of backyard allotted to the rowhouse, and most of our neighbors filled those spaces with hibachi charcoal grills and aluminum folding lawn chairs with colored nylon webbing. Adjacent to the living room was a kitchen with a small bar and a couple of stools where I remember my parents arguing loudly about the bills. The only serious allergic reaction that I experienced occurred following a second DTaP booster (to prevent tetanus, diphtheria, and whooping cough in young children), which was given at the wrong interval by mistake. After Mom ice packed it, the swelling of the injected arm gradually subsided in a day or two. In later years, I developed allergies to penicillin and to sulfa drugs like Bactrim, which once caused giant hives to break out on my body from head to toe until the drug cleared out of my system several days later.

After about three years in Centreville, my parents separated, divorced, and quickly remarried. Dad kept the townhouse in northern Virginia, and my brother and I moved to the southside of Richmond with my mother and her new husband Don. Dad drove down to see us every two weekends or so, a two-hour trip one-way. When we visited Centreville, he had us ride in the tiny hatchback of his Datsun 240Z. He chain-smoked most of the way but mercifully cracked the driver's side window to help clear second-hand smoke. Despite my asthma and other allergies, he smoked in the house too. Perhaps he regarded asthma as a psychological condition, as did many people in the 1970s. On weekends when we weren't around, he and his wife Dale raced sprint carts and auto-crossed their Datsun Zs. A capable driver, he would sometimes when I suffered fits of wheezing and shortness of breath in Centreville, motor around town while I lay in the back seat on my side. I found the movement of the car oddly comforting, and on those occasions at least, he forwent the cigarettes. It couldn't have been much fun for him having a sick little kid around; he had always hoped one of his boys would become an athlete. Instead, we're all pretty nerdy.

-◊-

My stepfather had transferred to the DuPont plant in Richmond, and he made a short commute every workday to the DuPont Fibers facility on Jefferson Davis Highway (Route 1) between Richmond and Petersburg. During the next few years, I cycled in and out of hospitals, usually staying for a week at a time. The typical trajectory of those asthma attacks went something like this: an encounter with an unknown allergen in the environment (perhaps at home, at school, at a friend's house, or outside) triggered bouts of sneezing and runny eyes. If that response continued for more than a few hours, wheezing and coughing commenced, which always worsened at night. Once lung congestion established itself, I began to wheeze and struggled to stay hydrated. When the chest got so tight that I couldn't take it anymore, I'd reluctantly ask to go to the doctor's office for shots of epinephrine, antihistamines, and steroids to get some relief. If I was lucky, Dr. Kellet, my pediatrician, would shoot me up, get me hydrated by forcing me to drink fluids, and send me home with a dose of Sus-Phrine (a long-acting form of epinephrine no longer produced).[39]

Those asthma attacks ranged from mild and infrequent to exceedingly severe, and the worst of them were characterized by choking and breathlessness, straining of the neck and chest muscles, a pale complexion and blue lips, a racing pulse, a sweaty face and body, and frightening sensations of suffocation. Even during the most extreme attacks, I hesitated to go to the doctor's office, because if an intravenous drip was needed to stay hydrated, there was better than a fifty-fifty chance that I'd be admitted to the pediatric ward. Hospital admission usually meant spending days and nights under an oxygen tent, attached by tubes and wires to medical machinery, enduring regular nebulizer breathing treatments and blood draws, and being woken up in the middle of the night to take medicines and to receive injections. I learned to expect cold rooms, drafty hospital clothes, patients coughing and moaning, x-ray machines that used large black plates framed in shiny steel, tasteless hospital food served on plastic cafeteria trays with divided compartments, and visits from well-meaning friends and family.

During one particularly fierce asthma attack, seared into my memory, we skipped the doctor's office and went straight to the Medical College of Virginia (now the VCU School of Medicine), a public hospital that at the time treated underserved communities in the Richmond area. The attack was so acute that Mom had to carry me through the parking garage, no easy feat given that I must have weighed 40 to 50 pounds. We entered a small, crowded waiting room filled with African American parents and their sick children. Because we were middle class, insured, and regarded as white, I was promptly admitted ahead of many of those waiting to be seen. That type of privilege, pervasive in the old South, fills me with sorrow that Virginia and other Southern states do so little to provide social services to the neediest people. Virginia did not expand Medicaid to cover 400,000 low-income residents until 2018.[40]

During these prolonged hospitalizations, which included days of being bombarded by medications injected directly into continual IV drips, I would sometimes hallucinate, and on at least one occasion leapt out of bed while still connected to the IV and flashing machines—and tried to fly. Another time, I had an out of body experience during which I observed myself from an alternate vantage point in the room: floating above my body and observing it, along with everything else, like a detached stranger. I'm not sure what synergy of drugs contributed to these experiences, some of which resemble the near-death reports discussed in the Conclusion, but the buildup of medications in the bloodstream over many days sometimes elicited such responses.

-◊-

Throughout the 1970s and early 1980s, food allergies remained poorly understood, including by people working in health care. In *Coping with Food Allergy* (1974), Dr. Claude Frazier noted that food allergy was an unusual disease that many people dismissed as a figment of the imagination or a symptom of hypochondria. "Even physicians," he wrote, "do not always understand the role it plays in a number of diseases," and "a good many parents even now are inclined to view their allergic child's symptoms with skepticism."[41] As a child moving towards adolescence with little understanding of food allergies, I only knew that tree nuts made me sick. Unfortunately, skepticism and ignorance by members of the medical community and general public meant that I didn't fully recognize those allergic reactions as indicative of extreme food allergies until the mid–1980s, when exposure necessitated prompt emergency medical care.

In retrospect, I experienced a series of allergic reactions to tree nuts during my pre-teen years that constituted a pattern of worsening responses, which culminated in the nearly fatal anaphylactic reaction to pecan that opens this chapter. Part of my struggle to understand that illness resulted from growing up at a time when food allergies were rare, but the encounters with nuts that follow illustrate the difficulties children and teens still face coping with food allergy as they are learning to negotiate social spaces of all sorts. Despite the allergic rhinitis (cough, stuffy nose, postnasal drip) that often led to hospitalizations for chronic asthma (itself a severe allergy symptom), I tried to live a normal life. I joined the Cub Scouts, a youth program run by the Boy Scouts of America for children from first to fifth grade, but my participation in that program occasioned two moments of profound social embarrassment.

In the neighborhood home of one scout leader, the host mother made milk and cookies for us after we completed a series of skill-building exercises that included how to start a campfire. The cookies must have contained tree nuts, for not long after eating several, I ran outside to vomit in the bushes. Discovering me retching in her yard, the hostess called my mother, who came to pick me up early, much to the amusement of the other boys. Another incident illustrates the social mortification that can occur to pre-teens suffering from the running nose, postnasal drip, and rhinitis that often accompanies childhood allergies to molds, pollens, and dust. During a pinewood derby race in a school auditorium, one of the mothers was talking with me amiably when she unexpectedly asked what was in the palm of my hand. I looked down at my left hand, which I thought was empty, and saw a wad of thick green mucus about the size of a half dollar—and promptly fled the room humiliated by the signs of sickness that my body had produced. For years afterward, I developed a poor self-image as a skinny nerdy kid with glasses and a long, snivelly nose large enough to hold a lot of snot.

The vomiting that was an early symptom of the food allergy gave way to worse reactions with each exposure to nuts. The difference between a food intolerance and a food allergy boils down to how the body handles an allergen. Food intolerance—a more common problem—involves metabolism rather than the immune system. When the body cannot adequately digest an offending food, it's often because of a chemical deficiency that produces symptoms such as abdominal cramping. Usually, some amount of the food can be tolerated before symptoms appear. By contrast, with a food allergy, the body's immune system recognizes the reaction-provoking substance—usually a protein—as a dangerous intruder and produces antibodies to stop the "invasion."[42] The mouth and lips swell, stomach cramps lead to vomiting, the skin often (though not always) breaks out in hives or rashes, the airways close. Because the only way to prevent these symptoms from manifesting is to practice complete avoidance of food antigens, the simple pleasure of eating becomes transformed into a painful, scary, and potentially fatal experience. In people like myself, *as little as one-fifth to one-five-thousandth of a teaspoon of an offending food can cause death*—with severe symptoms occurring in as little as five to fifteen minutes.[43]

As a kid, I only knew that I didn't like nuts and instinctively learned to avoid foods containing them because they made me sick, like the marshmallow ambrosia with walnuts and mixed fruit served by Nannie Nitti at holiday gatherings. When the ambrosia didn't make me vomit, eating even a small amount of it created what I can only describe as a blockage that felt like a fist where the esophagus meets the stomach. It made swallowing difficult, a sensation that could last for a couple of hours or more. During that time, I would lie down or hover over a toilet spitting out thick phlegm and hoping to throw up. Sometimes, those symptoms were accompanied by difficulty breathing and swelling of the lips and tongue. Like many boys fighting respiratory illness, I just wanted to run and play outside without collapsing into a wheezing mess. On the other hand, asthma provided a good excuse to avoid gym at school, and it kept me out of classes where known allergens were being used. I once waited outside of a classroom door while my peers experimented with mothballs and Bunsen burners. As a result of such avoidance behaviors, I experienced some bullying at school, but more debilitating was the psychology of illness, and the self-identification with allergies, that helped turn me into a rather solitary and bookish fellow, spoiled by his mother and strong-willed.

-◊-

Around the time that I turned nine or ten years old, my father transferred from the Centreville lab in Northern Virginia to the central laboratory in Richmond. He and my stepmother bought a modest contemporary home in Chesterfield County, ten miles from my mother and stepfather's place in sleepy Chester. Parceled in 1749 from Henrico County, Chesterfield County includes the site of the Henricus settlement founded in 1611 by English naval commander and deputy-governor Sir Thomas Dale for the Virginia Colony. Prior to the American Revolution, well-heeled travelers stopped for food and accommodation at the Half Way House in North Chesterfield between Richmond and Petersburg.

Dad's new wood-stained home, located four miles from the Half Way House and eight miles from the site of the Henricus settlement, sat midway down a neighborhood block that dead-ended near Crooked Branch Creek. That creek ran near a set of power lines (now a roadway), and together they created borders of a large play area that provided endless diversion to us kids. In our age of cell phones and Amber Alerts it may be difficult to imagine, but in the early 1980s older children generally wandered freely without much parental supervision. We were "latchkey kids" who went to school in the morning and came back in the afternoon to empty homes because our parents were working. That arrangement gave us plenty of time to make mischief of the useful and not-so-useful sort.

Living the Food-Allergic Life

Built in 1978 and located in the middle of a steep neighborhood block, Dad's house was situated near the rear of a narrow third-of-an-acre lot graded downward toward the street. Out back, a small fenced-in yard contained a few oak trees. The A-frame construction and dark brown wood siding accentuated a long roofline that sloped downward from its apex, like an upside-down checkmark. The attached garage in front of the house, with its symmetrical roofline, gave the home an almost Asian flare. The front steps led up to a small porch protected by a high, angled overhang. Inside, a linoleum floor designed to look like planks of wood ran like an oval racetrack around the kitchen and the stairs leading up to the second floor. At opposite ends of the kitchen, a living room and a dining room with a bay window.

The television, a blinking idol to commerce and entertainment, was always on when anyone in the house was awake, and it made the living room a central gathering point for meals. Veneer wood paneling ran three feet up the walls of the living room, and above it, off-white wallpaper with vertical green stripes reached to the ceiling. On the far wall, to the left of the television, an oddly-shaped bear rug—in orange. For a while, a pair of matching orange lava lamps completed the "décor." Upstairs, two tiny bedrooms lay to the right of the landing, and to the left, a master bedroom and slanted storage area under the pitched roof. The bedroom that Paul and I shared included a window that opened onto the garage roof, which was a great boon once we learned to open it, step out onto the roof, hang off the side of the garage, and drop to the ground below when we wanted to sneak out.

In that house, at around ten years of age, it became clear that I would have to figure out how to live with a dangerous food allergy at a time when many food products did not include accurate lists of ingredients. Dale occasionally baked cakes and cookies and once asked me to grind walnuts in a small nut grinder. It had a yellow plastic funnel-shaped top, a hand crank, and a glass container for collection. I sat at the laminate dinner table between the kitchen and television set while Dale worked behind me near the oven. When she returned to check on my progress, she found my hands, arms, neck, and face covered in hives. After vomiting cookies at the Cub Scout meeting and feeling sick following Nannie's ambrosia, I knew better than to eat any of the walnuts, but getting hives from just grinding them marked an important stage in the onset of more severe food allergies. From inhaling the dust of the ground walnuts, hives also appeared inside my mouth. I had a dentist appointment that day and recall being embarrassed about the staff seeing those swellings. It never occurred to me that one day this food allergy would become life threatening and transform my relationship to food forever. No one ever mentioned anaphylaxis, and I knew nothing about the speed at which it could kill.

The second allergic response to tree nuts in this house took place many years later. My brother Tony (nine years younger than me to the day and a happy consequence of Dad's second marriage) still has memories of it, though he was quite young at the time. Due to the complex interfamily dynamics that often accompany divorces and remarriages, and a certain emotional and intellectual distance from my father, this episode is difficult to recount even decades later. I cannot remember how the conversation between me and Dad started, but it became heated when he gave expression to a theory that my allergy to nuts (and by implication other allergic illnesses) were "all in my head." Under any circumstances, it's devastating for a sick child to be told by a parent that his illness is self-created, even though people at the time held similar views about asthma and food allergies—and, to be fair, one finds instances of anxiety and depression on both sides of my family.

Some years later, I had a friend named Mark, a nerdy asthmatic kid like me, whose mother (a single parent) "treated" his asthma by making him sit in the bedroom alone to "calm down." In *Coping with Food Allergy*, Claude Frazier recounts meeting a boy in his teens with a barrel chest, indicative of asthma of a long duration, who was clearly having an attack. The boy's father, an athletic coach, believed that his son's illness was emotional in origin, and he forced him to participate in many sports. Two weeks later, that young man died in the hospital.[44] Perhaps coming to the same conclusion as this coach, my father determined to test his hypothesis, and he asked me to close my eyes. I stood across from the stove facing the refrigerator, eyes tightly shut, when I heard the freezer door open. Some rustling of plastic bags ensued followed by a request to open my mouth. On my tongue, my father placed a large uncut almond, which I held there for a few seconds—and thankfully did not chew or swallow. I recall its cylindrical shape, like a large teardrop, and its coldness.

After a few seconds, I spit the curious object out, opened my eyes, and was furious to discover a whole almond. Profoundly upset that my Dad would experiment on me, I ran upstairs to the hallway bathroom in tears and rinsed out my mouth, but it was too late. My tongue, throat, and lips started to tingle and itch, and then the swelling began. The tongue expanded so much it no longer fit in my mouth. That fist-in-the-gut feeling returned, and I started drooling. After ten or fifteen minutes, I went downstairs to show my father the "psychological" reaction that his experiment had elicited. Dale thought to get me some Benadryl and the reaction abated in about two hours. Even after seeing the consequences of his experimentation, Dad continued to smoke in the house and in his cars—even though all three of his kids have allergies. And there were always nuts in the house when I stayed with him, often out in the open, and within reach. That fact makes it more difficult to explain how I could eat a pecan chocolate chip cookie at his place as an adult without *carefully* reading the ingredients, but it only takes one moment of carelessness to create a life-threatening situation.

-◊-

The term "allergy," derived from the Greek words *allos* (other) and *ergos* (work), was coined around 1907, and it refers to an "altered" reaction of the immune system that follows prior exposures to an allergen.[45] When the body is not reacting to an antigen, people with asthma, allergic rhinitis, and food allergies can generally go about their daily lives normally. Sure, I wake up almost every morning with postnasal drip and experience several bouts of sneezing per day, but before albuterol inhalers and corticosteroid nasal sprays, I could predict the onset of rainy weather based on hay fever-like symptoms. In comparison to anaphylaxis, those allergic responses are a nuisance, though as a pre-teen and teen they made me socially awkward: the constant sniveling, the stuffy nose that promoted heavy mouth breathing, the front jeans pocket full of Kleenex.

In middle school, my study habits became more focused. I answered questions in class, carried assorted pens in front shirt pockets like my scientist Dad, and brought gifts to generous teachers. I recall from those years plastic black-framed glasses, tan slacks, crocodile shirts, and thick brown hair parted to the side like my father's. In between the annual and biennial hospitalizations that defined this part of my life, I played in the woods, jumped through piles of raked leaves in the fall, rode bicycles to the local convenience store to buy candy and cola-flavored Slurpees, swam at the local pool, and played little league baseball (despite my slight build and poor endurance). Much of the time, I managed those activities with minimal interference from allergies, though there were exceptions.

We used to roam freely in the large field behind Mom and Don's house near Thomas Dale High School in Chester. Every summer, it filled with tall grasses and wildflowers, and we explored several old barns in various states of dilapidation on the property. My brother Paul and I climbed amid ruins of grey weathered boards looking for square hand-forged nails used to build tobacco curing and pack barns during the mid-to-late nineteenth century. Cure barns usually contained tier poles, supported by posts and cross beams on which tobacco leaves were hung to be air or fire cured. Pack barns, which might be partially log-constructed or wood-framed, provided space for tobacco leaf processing, storing, grading, and bundling. Prior to the Civil War, the onerous work of tobacco (and cotton) cultivation and processing fell to slaves. In the postbellum South, black and white sharecroppers or tenant farmers took on those tasks. Wandering among those fields, we discovered one day a litter of kittens amid barn remains. Not seeing a mother cat around, we concluded that they were abandoned, and we each brought a kitten home, holding it in our arms during the walk back through the high grass. Infatuated with the kittens, we ignored our running eyes, sneezing, and my wheezing, which prompted Mom to order us into bathtubs and to wash our clothes. We thought we had "rescued" the kittens, but cat dander triggers allergic responses on par with exposure to mold and mildew infestation. Today, my brother Paul has the more serious allergy to cats.

-◊-

By my second year of high school, something surprising happened. I began to outgrow some environmental allergies and the cycle of hospitalization that marked my youth gradually ceased. A 1984 yearbook photo shows a pubescent boy with glasses too large for his face, short straight hair, and a black pullover shirt that unsnapped from the left shoulder to reveal a triangle-shaped patch of gray fabric underneath (a fashion inspired by the astounding success of the album *Thriller* two years earlier). In adolescence, I found a small measure of popularity when I started to hang out with the "cool kids." Sure, I had to carry a blue inhaler in the front pocket of my jeans, but an untucked oversized shirt covered it up.

I could manage the allergic asthma by hitting an albuterol inhaler during the day and throughout the night, when symptoms were worse, but the allergies to tree nuts began to intensify. That escalation came at a difficult time. Research shows that teenagers with severe food allergies engage in greater degrees of "risky eating" than adults, and they more frequently fail to seek prompt treatment after exposure. Peer pressure, dating, kissing, drinking alcohol, increased risk taking, and the reluctance to carry bulky epinephrine auto-injectors all contribute to higher incidence of fatal anaphylaxis among pre-teens and teens.[46] Untreated or poorly managed asthma may make anaphylaxis worse due to wheezing and swelling of lung tissue, so adolescents with food allergies should properly manage their asthma and asthmatic symptoms.[47]

Like many Americans then and now, I began to date in high school. While I knew enough to recognize the need to avoid eating tree nuts, I failed to always maintain necessary levels of vigilance. During my junior year, a youthful propensity for romance led to a frightening allergic response—and my first dance with anaphylaxis. It started after school at Angela's house in the Salem Woods Lake community of North Chesterfield. Built during the late 1970s, Salem Woods Lake featured small one-story ranch and Cape Cod style homes with uncovered brick porches and pastel-colored vinyl siding. To the north, an elementary and middle school sat side-by-side, the cookie-cutter homes situated below them like strings of a puppeteer's marionette.

Angela's dark hair, freckles, and green eyes framed a distinctive diminutive nose that flattened slightly in the middle. Like mine, her parents worked during the day. One afternoon, we hung out at her place for an hour or two after school. As I got up to leave, she brought out a blue plate piled with homemade chocolate chip cookies and asked me to try one. Without thinking, I did so, and immediately felt an unpleasant tingling sensation on my tongue and in the back of my throat. When I asked about ingredients, she told me that the cookies contained ground almonds—which is why I did not notice them initially. A bit frightened, I drove to the small home off Beach Road where I lived with Mom, a distance of about 11 miles (or 16 to 17 minutes). On the way, I began to have difficulty breathing.

By the time I arrived, my tongue no longer fit in my mouth. Frightened and embarrassed, I locked myself in the hallway bathroom, monitored my condition in the mirror, and waited for the reaction to subside. My mother, single again, was working fulltime as a nurse and commuted to Charlottesville to complete a master's degree at University of Virginia. I was still stationed in the bathroom with the door locked when she got home. When she learned what had happened, she convinced me to open the door. As I did so, she grew alarmed and drove me immediately to a private health care franchise, open seven days a week from morning to night, which was closer than the hospital emergency room.

In addition to the absurdly swollen tongue hanging out of my mouth, I was wheezing and drooling, and for that reason was seen immediately. "Oh my God," the doctor exclaimed when he saw my face—a response that compounded my worry. But the good man hit me with a couple of injections of epinephrine, and within a few hours, I was released from care. Unfortunately, on the return ride, I experienced rebound anaphylaxis, in which symptoms will abate for a while, but then suddenly recur. Most rebound (biphasic) responses take place within eight hours of exposure, but they can be delayed up to 72 hours. There's little consensus on an optimal period of observation for patients treated for anaphylaxis, either.[48] In the passenger seat of Mom's gray Mazda RX7, I suddenly became extremely short of breath. Once home, she had to phone for an ambulance. A nurse by training, she calmly informed the dispatcher that I was entering anaphylactic shock. When the ambulance arrived, we rode to the emergency room, where I was hit with more epinephrine and antihistamines. I don't fault the first private medical center for not keeping me longer after the first wave of allergic response, but anyone with anaphylaxis should be mindful of the possibility of rebounds.

-◊-

In the 1990s, researchers estimated that approximately 30,000 Americans rushed to emergency rooms every year for treatment of food allergies, but more recent studies suggest that figure is closer to 200,000 (including 90,000 for probable anaphylaxis).[49] Hundreds of them die every year. One would think that after so many terrible encounters with tree nuts, I would have been more vigilant, but four years later, in 1989, I ate what looked like a piece of pure milk chocolate. It was flavored with pralines, and I went into shock again. I had only just managed to graduate from high school two years earlier. With low marks and facing a family expectation to complete a college degree, I enrolled at Richard Bland College, a two-year school established in 1960 by the Virginia General Assembly as a branch of the College of William and Mary. While commuting to Petersburg to take courses and raise my GPA, I worked part-time waiting tables, selling clothes in the mall, and stocking grocery store shelves. I transferred to Virginia Commonwealth University in Richmond the following year.

To save money, I lived with Dad, Dale, and Tony and commuted north to Richmond on the Interstate 95 corridor. Dad paid for tuition and books, as was agreed when he and Mom divorced, but other expenses associated with school and later housing were mine to manage. To pay for a car, gas, clothes, pocket money, and other obligations, I worked about twenty hours a week, took classes fulltime, and later played guitar in a local band. Richmond City differed considerably from the suburbs south of the James River where I grew up, and the economic and racial disparities that characterized it at the time were but one manifestation of that variance. Situated about 50 miles northwest of the site of Jamestown, the first permanent English settlement in North America, Richmond became an economic center prior to the Revolutionary War. In 1775, Patrick Henry delivered his famous "Give Me Liberty or Give Me Death" speech against the Tax Act at St. John's Church on East Broad Street, and troops under the command of turncoat Benedict Arnold went on a rampage and burned the city in 1781.

Shockoe Bottom, east of downtown near the James River, became the second largest slave trading center in the nation during the antebellum period. Traders sold hundreds of thousands of men, women, and children at Shockoe Bottom into slavery throughout the South. That cruel legacy still haunts the city, as does its decision to serve as the second capital of the Confederacy from May 1861 to April 1865. The Union's nine-month siege of Petersburg led by General Ulysses S. Grant severed crucial Confederate supply lines to General Robert E. Lee's army and forced his retreat from Richmond and Petersburg. As they fled, the Confederates set fire to bridges, warehouses, an armory, and the flames spread out of control and burned a quarter of Richmond's buildings. After a failed attempt to reach the railway at Lynchburg for supplies, Lee surrendered at Appomattox Court House on April 9, 1865.

I commuted to Richmond for school and work during the late 1980s and early 1990s, and for me at least, the legacy of slavery, segregation, and racism in the city became apparent. The Thirteenth Amendment freed African Americans from slavery and involuntary servitude, and they moved off rural farms to urban centers like Richmond. When Reconstruction ended in 1877, white Democrats began to regain control of state legislatures and governorships across the South. They kept former slaves from owning property and systematically denied them the same rights as white Americans using Jim Crow laws to enforce segregation. The *State* newspaper in Richmond once proclaimed that the "best government in the world" could be ensured only by the "rule of the best people," meaning white property owners.[50] Richmond segregated its public school system in 1869; a convict system dispatched blacks convicted of petty crimes to hard labor (while whites could pay fines); black schools and public libraries operated without sufficient funding (despite the pretense of "separate but equal" facilities); and the state imposed poll taxes, understanding clauses, and literacy tests for all voters to limit black turnout.[51] Jim Crow laws remained in effect in Virginia until passage of the Civil Rights Act of 1964 and the Voting Rights Act of 1965.

-◊-

As I became more familiar with the city, it became clear that Richmond remained highly segregated. The area west of Virginia Commonwealth University marked the start of the historic Fan district—a large, walkable, upper–middle class inner-city neighborhood developed between 1890 and 1930 that took its name from the way streets radiated outward west of downtown starting at Monroe Park. Restaurants, shops, and elegantly appointed Edwardian and Revival style homes painted in a variety of muted shades (blues, beiges, light greens, and grays) grace the Fan's tree-lined avenues. On one of its leading thoroughfares, Monument Avenue, once stood towering bronze statues of Confederates J.E.B. Stuart, Robert E. Lee, Jefferson Davis, and Stonewall Jackson. Students tended to occupy the large houses converted to apartments closest to campus, but sections of the Fan further west attracted old Richmond money to fine homes and townhomes and channeled financial support to institutions such as the Virginia Museum of Fine Arts and the United Daughters of the Confederacy. Carytown, adjacent to the Museum district, catered to a mostly upper-class clientele—with the exception of dollar movie nights at the historic Byrd Theater and a few pizza joints.

The affluent whites who populated the Fan District were surrounded to the south by the working-class neighborhood of Oregon Hill and to the northwest by the former industrial district of Scott's Addition with its factories and warehouses, minor league baseball park, and local businesses (including Binswanger Glass and Curles Neck Dairy and Bar). The predominantly African American neighborhoods of Church Hill, Jackson Ward, and Gilpin north and east of downtown became sites of concentrated poverty, violent crime, and drug trafficking and made Richmond the second deadliest city per capita in the nation in 1994 (with 161 homicides). Amid a renewed spike in murders in recent years, city leaders continue to seek remedies for Richmond's legacy of segregation and racism by hiring more black police officers, improving economic conditions, and providing educational opportunities for residents in economically disadvantaged areas.

As proof that I entered Virginia Commonwealth University a glum and materialistic 19-year-old business major (with an intended focus on information systems), one of my assignments in English 101 was to keep a journal. The pages of that journal have sustained damage over the years from improper storage, but the writing is still legible. The entry from January 18, 1989, opens: "I have been preoccupied with death for several weeks now. What happens to us when we die? Is there really something else out there waiting to retrieve our souls? I'm really not that religious of a person and don't really believe in a god." This almost unrecognizable self asks, "Is death the blackness of not existing," before he expresses a hope "to remain a little bit longer" on this earth—because he really wants to buy a Porsche 911 Carrera! These days, I feel lucky to drive a six-year-old black Ford Fiesta with a six-speed transmission.

The second journal entry dated February 13, full of syntactical errors and misspellings, begins: "Today was a fucked up day! I have a severe allergy to nuts and came in contact with them at Thalhimers candy store and had to be rushed to the emergency room." A more accurate rendering of that event would be that I was walking through a shopping mall with my buddy Mike and his friend Bill with whom I share an interest in classic cars. Mike, a slim, bearded native Virginian with a distinctive drawl, stopped in front of the Godiva chocolate stand and bought three pieces of candy. He offered one to me, what looked like a small square of milk chocolate called a "praline." Being foolish, I had no idea that pralines, made by boiling nuts (often pecans, almonds, or hazelnuts) in sugar, frequently filled chocolate candies. In those days, I still ate plain Hershey's milk chocolate bars, as well as cakes and cookies that I could determine were nut-free, and I didn't carry epinephrine auto-injectors. Reflecting upon the careless way that I thoughtlessly accepted the praline, and Angela's chocolate chip cookie years earlier, this situation demonstrates why adolescents and young adults with severe food allergies are at greater risk of anaphylaxis.

Immediately sensing the familiar itching in the mouth and tongue that often, though not always, signals the onset of an allergic reaction, I experienced a sense of impending doom similar to that at my father's house twelve years later. I told Mike and Bill that I needed to get to a hospital, and we walked briskly out of the mall, into the parking lot, and headed for the car. On the way, my breathing became short, and I started to turn blue. "Hurry, please hurry," I remember begging Bill, who was driving. Admitted immediately upon arrival, my journal records slipping into bronchospasms and receiving several injections of adrenaline and Benadryl, along with multiple breathing treatments. For some inexplicable reason, Mike and Bill were admitted into the treatment room, which caused me additional anxiety—and it meant they had to watch an anaphylactic reaction unfold. I sat on the edge of a hospital bed, legs dangling off the side, my shirt off, while they helplessly watched me struggle for air. "I have lived with asthma my whole life," I wrote the next day, "but have never had such a reaction. Pulling for every breath, literally."

For about 45 minutes to an hour, I felt on the edge of passing out until the doctors and nurses managed to get the reaction under control. Mike, on whom watching my agony made an indelible impression, told me later that he didn't think I would make it. But after some time, a young nurse assured me, "you're not going to die." Her declaration reduced some of the fear assailing me, and her prognosis proved correct. I was released from care hours later. On the drive home, I watched for signs of rebound anaphylaxis, which never came. "I wonder if I would have died," I mused in the journal, "if I just would have blacked out and ceased to exist?" The subsequent entry penned less than two weeks later, on my twentieth birthday, suggests that coming that close to death had a clarifying effect on my perspective and attitude. I expressed gratitude for the gift of an electric guitar and small transistor amp that my girlfriend Susan had given to me for my birthday. I've never been able to properly thank her, but that gift has filled my life with music. Post-anaphylaxis, I also better appreciated family, friends, the opportunity to go to school—though that sense of appreciation seems to have been temporary, for the following month, I was complaining about a lack of meaningful course content.

After completing that semester, I continued journaling for a year, and those scribblings reveal an increasing frustration with the business curriculum. By October 1989, I'd started reading Plato, Emerson, Freud, Erik Erikson and Carl Sagan, and listening to Mozart and Led Zeppelin. Soon thereafter, I found myself in Walter's world literature course, and still recall the profound impact that William Blake's poetry and artwork made on me. The net effects of those adventures in ideas made me "very disheartened with the prospect of a business career." This "dark night of the soul" was punctuated with references to depression and oppressive feelings about the plight of humanity and the environment. By spring 1990, I recorded feeling "very pleased" at the prospect of the literature, philosophy, and psychology classes that I had signed up for— though they did little to move me toward graduation. My band, Floating Well, developed musically and provided an opportunity to write chord progressions and lyrics. By my twenty-first birthday, I had started collecting book ideas, though it would be more than two decades before I would write or publish one.

Somewhere I found the courage to switch my major to English education and then to general studies, so that I could design my own coursework ("religious and philosophical dimensions in literature") and avoid the college foreign language requirement. During the fall semester, I began to raise a mediocre GPA by taking classes such as early American Literature, Islam, Zen Buddhism, Creative Writing, and Psychology and Religion. I moved to a small one-bedroom flat on the second floor of a Monument Avenue apartment building after graduation, started a master's program in English at Virginia Commonwealth, and continued to wait tables and play music at small venues around town. Although passed over for a graduate teaching assistantship, I worked part-time at the James Branch Cabell Library as a graduate assistant in the reference department.

I contemplated enrolling in a library science program, but Mom suggested a career in teaching, and to test those waters, I began substituting for Chesterfield County Public Schools. Within a year, I had filled-in for kindergarten to twelfth grade teachers in subjects ranging from physical education to mathematics. A long-term substitute opportunity in what was then called special education helped me to discover an unexpected talent in the classroom. After many challenging moments, including one in which I lost control of a rowdy group of students and another in which a kid just turned and bolted for the fences during an outdoor activity, I decided that teaching college might prove a better fit. A few months prior to graduating with a master's degree, the band broke up before playing a gig that I booked at the Flood Zone in 1995 opening for the enormously successful Dave Matthews Band. That great disappointment encouraged me to start answering advertisements in a TESOL newsletter for English teachers overseas. During the next two years, I would teach English language and writing courses at Kyungnam University in South Korea—and during that time had another troubling encounter with tree nuts in an unexpected place.

CHAPTER TWO

Departures into the Unknown
-or-
This Beautiful World

"Avoiding danger is no safer in the long run than outright exposure. The fearful are caught as often as the bold."—Helen Keller, *Let Us Have Faith* (1940)

"To travel is worth any cost or sacrifice."—Elizabeth Gilbert, *Eat Pray Love* (2010)

-◊-

Among the reasons I found to be apprehensive about teaching in the Far East: I had never traveled or lived abroad, did not speak Korean, knew little about Korean culture, and had limited teaching experience. Having a food allergy compounded these worries, and the bit of language learning that I undertook before departing focused on parroting common phrases (most carefully those related to food) from two audio cassettes purchased at a local bookstore. I brought a couple of epinephrine auto-injectors with me, but they usually expire in a year or so and were expensive without medical insurance (about $100 each at the time). I never saw epinephrine auto-injectors in the local Korean pharmacies, as food allergies were relatively uncommon among Koreans in the mid-to-late 1990s. On the other hand, albuterol and other allergy medications were readily available without a prescription and were much cheaper than in the United States.

I applied to Kyungnam University, a regional institution enrolling about 15,000 students, because they had advertised for master's prepared instructors who could teach English as a Second Language (ESL) to first-year college students. Those selected had to also teach one class for their for-profit language institute (*hagwon*) that offered children and adults in the community an opportunity to learn another language. The most important qualifications, I found out later, were the master's degree in English (or related field) from an accredited university—and being a native English speaker. After teaching sections of the same first-year course for the ESL program, I moved to the English department the following year, where I first learned to teach literature and writing. During those two years, I edited several books translated into English for Korean and Japanese colleagues and published a first peer-reviewed journal article (on William Blake and Ch'an Buddhism in the *Journal of Chinese Philosophy*).

For someone right out of graduate school, it seemed miraculous to be living in Masan, a coastal city in the southern part of the Korean peninsula approximately 28 miles from Busan. With a small efficiency apartment, a salary of $18,000 per year (paid in Korean *won*), and long summer and winter breaks included, it was a difficult offer to pass up, even given the risks of eating in a foreign country. Quite accidently, South Korea turned out to be a good choice for someone with a tree nut allergy—so long as I avoided bakeries and desserts in restaurants and cafés. Staple foods include rice, vegetables, and meat (chicken, beef, pork, fish, seafood). Standardized recipes for popular dishes made daily life easier, but the extensive use of red chilies could sometimes cause a burning sensation on the tongue and lips that mimicked the onset of anaphylaxis. The practice of grilling directly on barbeque restaurant tables meant that I could find a meal almost anywhere by ordering a bowl of white rice, a side of *kimchi* (fermented cabbage dressed in red pepper), and a serving of meat. Water chestnuts appear in many dishes including *samgyetang* (ginseng chicken soup), and they concerned me at the time. I avoided them, but later learned that water chestnuts are the tubers of a water plant—not tree nuts.

There also existed less tasty and less healthy alternatives to traditional Korean food, including American fast-food restaurants like McDonald's and Kentucky Fried Chicken, as well as a plethora of Korean pizza joints featuring pies with unusual toppings such as maraschino cherries (the preserved sweet kind sold in jars of red liquid) and kernels of corn. Because of its proximity to the coast, people in Masan eat a lot of seafood, and I remember liking the fresh-water eel barbecued at one local hotspot. Reading packaged food labels in Korea proved a challenge even with a dictionary, and in any case, the accurateness of ingredient lists was dubious at best (one of many things that has changed for the better in the last 20+ years). When ordering in restaurants, it always helped to have a Korean friend to parse menus and to ask questions. Once a packaged food such as ramen noodles, or dishes in a particular restaurant, proved "safe," I tended to stick with those choices, even after they became boring.

In truth, I was extremely careless for someone with a potentially fatal food allergy who had survived anaphylaxis twice, especially given the tendency for my reactions to worsen with each exposure. Mom would occasionally mail an epinephrine auto-injector to me in Korea and later China, but I rarely carried them, except when traveling. Nor did I wear medical alert jewelry, which would have informed doctors in foreign countries about my condition, since it was possible that I could be in shock and disoriented by the time I made it to an emergency room. Yet, aside from one incidence of food poisoning, and the annual health examinations required to stay in the country on a work visa, I managed to steer clear of hospitals in South Korea. Though given little occasion to avail myself of it, the medical care I received was always competent, and I may have never felt as good in my life as when I made a foray into traditional herbal medicines. Nonetheless, in moving to South Korea, I knew that I was taking a considerable risk, but the opportunity to gain university teaching experience and to learn about East Asian culture firsthand seemed worth it. My reckless eating overseas, however, caught up with me during a three-day visit to Kyoto, Japan.

-◊-

For many expat teachers, one of the boons of working abroad is the ability to travel to otherwise far-flung countries during summer and winter breaks, for weeks, sometimes months, at a time. Although I managed to visit Thailand, China, Japan, and the island of Bali in Indonesia, those trips always gave rise to deep-seated fears about finding nut-free meals, fears which were compounded by the challenges of learning stock phrases in the local language, figuring out the value of the currency, familiarizing myself with the dangers faced by tourists (such as thievery), and avoiding transportation accidents or getting hopelessly lost. Before the advent of GPS and smartphones, we clung to guidebooks and phrasebooks to get around, to find accommodations, and to conduct rudimentary conversations. I tried to avoid any food containing nuts by eating in places where I could see ingredients, including roadside food stalls. Fortunately, I have never been a "foodie" and always eat to live—rather than living to eat. From my vantage point, any meal that does not kill me is a good one!

The seven thousand miles that I put between myself and Richmond cured heartbreak over Susan and the breakup of the band, and after about six months in South Korea, I met a young woman about my age who worked as a nutritionist for the university. Employing a common honorific that we used to address unmarried Korean women with whom we worked, my friends and I called her Ms. Seong. She had small, almond-shaped eyes, a petite nose, and short dark hair, and wore thick-framed glasses. Though shy, she possessed an adventurous spirit. Dating a *kojangi*, a big-nose person (i.e., a foreigner) took guts in the conservative and inward-looking Hermit Kingdom, and her boss despised the idea of our dating. Our relationship eventually cost Ms. Seong her job, and though she once brought me home to meet her parents, it was clear that they would not support our relationship. Because a 26-year-old unmarried woman in South Korea risked becoming a "Christmas cake girl" (someone past marriage age), her parents insisted that she go on arranged dates—a common practice in the country— while we were together.

One spring, we decided to visit Kyoto, Japan, even though Ms. Seong really wanted to tour the United States. We had planned to introduce her to my family, and my father wrote an invitation letter on her behalf, but she was denied a visa for not having at least $10,000 in her bank account. (Today, South Koreans can visit the United States without a visa for up to 90 days.) Disappointed, we opted instead for the "Land of the Rising Sun." Kyoto excited me because I had taken a Zen Buddhism class at Virginia Commonwealth with Cliff Edwards, who had studied at Daitoku-ji, a training center for the Rinzai sect. Kyoto, once known as Heian, became the imperial capital of Japan in 794. The 6,000-acre planned city borrowed its basic grid layout from the Tang dynasty city of Changan with its gated walls, imperial palace compound, pagodas, temples, and markets. A golden age of arts, literature, and high culture flourished in Kyoto from the time of the city's founding until 1185.

Two of the best accounts of courtly life during the Heian Era (794–1185) were penned by Japanese women. Lady Murasaki's *Tale of Genji* (c. 1021), sometimes regarded as the world's first novel, recounts the life and amours of Prince Genji, the dashing and talented son of a Japanese emperor.[1] Sei Shonagon's *The Pillow Book* (1002) provides a more personal account of life in the Heian court through a notebook-like collection of lists, poems, pithy anecdotes, character sketches, descriptions of nature, and love letters. Kyoto remained the capital of Japan until 1868 when the imperial household moved to Tokyo. Although little of Kyoto's historical architecture predates the 17th century (because the predominantly wooden structures did not withstand fire, war, or earthquake), the Allied Forces spared the city the worst ravages of the bombing campaign during World War II. The United States had considered targeting Kyoto, a haven for Japanese intellectuals, with an atomic bomb toward the end of World War II, but Secretary of War Henry Stimson insisted that the city be removed from a list of possible targets.[2] As a result, hundreds of wonderful Shinto shrines, Buddhist temples, imperial palaces, and splendid gardens in Kyoto—some dating back centuries—survived.

For these reasons, I thought Kyoto, situated in a fertile valley surrounded by the rolling hills of the Tamba highlands, would make a great getaway—and I figured on handling the problem of finding nut-free meals by keeping it simple: rice, ramen noodles, and occasionally American fast food. The flight from Busan to Osaka took little more than an hour, and the train from Osaka to Kyoto another 60 minutes or so. From there, we caught the rail line to the Arashiyama district famous for bamboo groves, sprawling Buddhist temples, pleasure boats, and elegant gardens. Assuming that we could find accommodations "on the fly" (as we did when traveling around South Korea), we failed to book hotels ahead of time. To our surprise, accommodations proved a challenge in the heavily touristed city, but fortunately we found a second-floor bedroom in a private home on our first night. I cannot remember whether the room was booked the following day, or whether we found it somewhat cramped, but the next morning we left with our backpacks, figuring that we would find another room while sightseeing.

On our second day in Japan, Ms. Seong wore a light white dress, a cream-colored baseball hat (no logo, worn backwards, askance), and reddish-brown leather ankle boots with olive green socks. We marveled together at the reflection of the Golden Pavilion in Mirror Pond, and its ten stone islands out of which pine trees miraculously grow, and the splendid wooden temples and shrines with graceful eaves that seem to float in the wind. We strolled through moss gardens and bamboo groves and sat quietly before rock gardens with sand raked in symmetrical patterns. We found Daitoku-ji, established by Zen Master Daito Kokushi in 1315, and toured its grounds. Arashiyama, on the western outskirts of Kyoto, has attracted visitors for centuries, so finding a hotel room that night proved almost impossible.

Just before nightfall, we walked past a posh traditional Japanese-style hotel with a vacancy. At $300 per night, it was well beyond my budget, but I carried a credit card for emergencies, and we gladly took it. Given the previous night's homestay, the room seemed especially opulent with its tatami mats and elegant carved wooden-frame doors finished with paper. The room fee included a traditional dinner and breakfast served in our room by women in kimonos who bowed before entering and leaving. That level of service remains beyond my expectation, and I don't enjoy the formality of it. I avoid fancy hotels and restaurants and the haute cuisine one finds in them, as such places are more likely to serve tree nuts. I made an exception, as I did with that praline chocolate at Thalhimers department store years earlier, when I decided to try some of the dishes set upon the folding lacquer table placed before us on the tatami.

Photos from that trip have survived and three of them were taken in that hotel room. The first shows a spacious living area overlooking a forest of trees. It was sparse, simple, and refined in the inimitable Japanese style, which writer Junichiro Tanizaki celebrated in his essay "In Praise of Shadows" (1933). When the dinner table was brought in, Ms. Seong seated herself on the floor in front of it, jubilant. She wore a light black V-neck sweater over a white dress. As I took the photo, she held both hands up at shoulder height and smiled widely, her lipstick the color of wet clay. Short bangs of hair fell in front of her eyes. On the table, just the accouterments for tea—even chopsticks had yet to appear. Near the window sat a single Western-style chair, and three light purple pillows rested in the corner. I stood up at my seat across from Ms. Seong to take the second picture, which shows a table full of delicate looking foods served in an attractive variety of lacquered dishes and saucers. Because neither of us spoke Japanese, we could not ask about ingredients.

As I stare now at that photo of the food on the table, I realize that the only thing that I should have taken was a wedge of melon, possibly the tempura vegetables, and the saki poured into small thimble-shaped cups. After walking all day though, we were hungry, and rice would be served last (since decorum prescribed first eating the dainty dishes). Not long into the meal, I remember cutting a small cube of tofu with my chopsticks. Allergists warn against trying to "test" a food for allergens by touching it, tasting it, or eating a tiny portion of it—and this is why. As soon as I put a bit of tofu into my mouth and swallowed, I knew from the tingling and burning that I had made another grave error in judgment and needed to get to a doctor quickly. Fortunately, the front desk staff spoke English, so we hurried out to the lobby, leaving an otherwise fine meal on the table. At reception, Ms. Seong quickly explained what had happened and asked for a doctor. A young man came out from the office behind the desk and drove us to a clinic (not a hospital emergency room).

Short of breath by the time we arrived, I was seen quickly, but with neither of us able to communicate in Japanese, we had to trust the doctor's judgment. He gave me several injections, and while they helped a bit, I continued to struggle to breathe. I was covered in hives and becoming pale. Perhaps because I had eaten so little of what we found out later was walnut tofu, I wasn't quite on the point of passing out. During previous dances with anaphylaxis, the inability to breathe was most terrifying. Halfway through this reaction, though, I became very calm inside and thought to myself, "it's okay to die now." I would have hated to leave Ms. Seong in a foreign country with a corpse to deal with, but she was bright and would make it home safely. Oddly, I wondered if my mother, who was on the other side of the world, knew that I was on the brink again (she didn't). The only other time that I felt that deep sense of peace that accompanies reconciliation to death was when the band hosted a Halloween party in a business warehouse full of highly flammable chemicals used in industrial flooring. Gradually realizing that one spark could cause a conflagration, I watched as people casually smoked around barrels of the stuff while we performed—and remember thinking "well, there are worse ways to go than playing music."

When repeated injections failed to halt the allergic reaction, I wrote (and probably misspelled) "Benadryl" for the Japanese doctor. Thankfully, he understood, adjusted my medications, and I started to feel better after several hours. Just after midnight, Ms. Seong and I took a cab back to the hotel. The serving staff, confused by our departure, had left the meal out thinking that we'd be hungry. Once they took it away, we pulled out the futons and slept on the tatami. The next morning, I took a third photo, from the same position as the first two, this time across a bento box breakfast that captures an utterly exhausted Ms. Seong: no makeup, eyes puffy from a night of crying, a sad—almost shocked—expression on her sullen face. A pair of blue jeans and a black t-shirt replaced the dress. She stares into space, probably pondering what she had witnessed the night before and mulling over the fragility of her boyfriend's health. Whenever we discussed that incident later, she always remarked on how little of the walnut tofu it took to trigger a reaction. Had I eaten more of it, the outcome might have been different, given that they probably could not have intubated me in that small clinic.

The next day, we returned to South Korea. Maybe because of the social pressure that Ms. Seong faced dating a foreigner, or because she didn't want to follow someone with an unpredictable illness overseas, or because she met someone else on the arranged dates, or because I misunderstood something about our relationship, we broke up months later—and I left for a teaching position in Shanghai, alone. Even so, I hope that this encounter with anaphylaxis has proven useful to her as a nutritionist.

-◊-

I had once joined a small group of fellow instructors (Jen, a future secondary teacher; Matt, who lived with the neurological consequences of a head injury; and Paul, a visual artist and cancer survivor) for a month-long trip through eastern China during the first summer in South Korea. We planned an adventurous itinerary that included Beijing, Shanghai, Nanjing, Guilin, Guangzhou, and Hong Kong—before returning to Shanghai to fly back to Masan. Backpacking through China on a budget in 1997 meant riding in trains, buses, vans, and taxis and staying at two-star hotels. I remember the train ride from Nanjing to Guilin being very inexpensive, but we had to stand for most of the 10-hour trip in Mao-era green and yellow train cars. Our fellow travelers sat on wooden benches and huddled around slab tables on which sat drinks, snacks, and sometimes baggage. The smell of urine and feces spread through the car whenever a bathroom door was opened. The Chinese passengers were friendly, and they let us sit down from time-to-time.

During those four weeks in China, we traveled approximately 2,000 miles without taking a flight. During our first stopover in Shanghai, a young woman name Estella who worked at the Shanghai Art Museum befriended me after a brief conversation about Chinese art. Our little group of English teachers continued to Guangzhou in southern China, and there we secured visas for Hong Kong—just a few days after the territory had been returned to China in 1997. After about four days in the former British colony, we returned to Shanghai. Shortly thereafter, Estella took me by train to see the Terra Cotta warriors in Xian. After I returned to South Korea, we stayed in touch via e-mail and post. When my second term contract at Kyungnam University was about to expire, I started looking for teaching positions elsewhere and began to prepare to apply to doctoral programs in literary studies back home. When she heard about those plans, the industrious Estella asked me for my résumé—and she faxed it to the foreign affairs offices of colleges and universities in Shanghai. A few weeks before finishing my last semester in Masan, I received a call from the Foreign Languages and Literatures Department at Fudan University with an offer to teach writing and American literature to undergraduates. I accepted with alacrity, signed the paperwork, secured a work visa, and booked a one-way ticket to Shanghai.

A respected institution of higher learning founded in 1905, six years before the fall of the Qing dynasty, Fudan enrolls some of the brightest students in the country. At that time, most undergraduates bunked six-to-a-room in unheated dormitories with a single bathroom per floor. Foreign faculty housing units, by contrast, had kitchenettes, a living room, one to three bedrooms (depending on the size of a visiting scholar's family), and heat in the winter—at least until 10 p.m. Most important for me, the local cuisine did not contain as many tree nuts as in other parts of the country. Exceptions existed, but one could *usually* see nuts in dishes (as opposed to being pureed in sauces or hidden in tofu). International chain restaurants and foreign supermarkets with product ingredients labeled in English provided an additional level of safety, but truth be told, during those four years in East Asia—I was incredibly lucky. I had acquired a "sweet tooth" from my father's side of the family, who always had fresh pastries (half-moons, eclairs, cannolis) from Harrison Bakery in Syracuse on hand—and not infrequently I ate Hostess cupcakes from the foreign grocery store for breakfast!

Although my salary in China amounted to just a few hundred dollars a month, faculty housing, roundtrip airfare, and a small travel stipend were included. By Chinese standards of the time, it was a good arrangement, but it meant foregoing pricey epinephrine auto-injectors during my stay, though I did carry Benadryl. Working with students at Fudan still ranks among the most meaningful experiences of my life, and the risks that I took moving to South Korea and China made me a better teacher, helped me to gain admission to graduate school, and allowed me to meet my bright and talented wife of more than twenty years. In spring 1999, during the final semester in China, I taught three classes and sat for the Graduate Record Exam (GRE) and the GRE subject test in literature in Shanghai twice to boost my scores.

When the doctoral program in English at University of Denver accepted me into their literary studies program with a teaching stipend, it meant leaving Shanghai for good. I remember walking down the steps of the foreign teacher's dormitory one afternoon with Arno, a French instructor at the university who lived with his girlfriend Sabine in the apartment above mine. A handsome fellow with a thin face, brownish-blonde hair, and a prominent nose, the overall impression Arno gave was one of youthful vitality, intelligence, and good taste. He was equally matched by Sabine, a beautiful dark-haired woman of Middle Eastern and European heritage who taught French at the university and studied Chinese.

As the semester drew to a close, several undergraduates asked me to participate in an event planned by students in the Foreign Language and Literature Department. They envisioned an international program that would showcase weddings as features of the languages and cultures they had studied. Their program included French, Chinese, and Korean wedding ceremonies highlighting divergent cultural approaches to the matrimonial ritual. A group of planners approached me after class and inquired if I would join the Chinese ceremony as a bridegroom. I agreed—on the condition that I could choose my own "bride," the woman, unbeknownst to my students, who inexplicably had agreed to marry the skinny fellow with the deadly food allergy a few weeks earlier.

The night of the ceremonies, Foreign Language and Literature Department students and their friends assembled in a large auditorium, festively decorated with bright paper banners for the occasion. Arno and Sabine, who several years later would wed in Europe, took the role of the French couple. Arno looked dashing in his tuxedo and Sabine lovely in her flowing white dress. As part of their ceremony, a black blindfold was placed over Arno's eyes, and then the students assembled a line of young women from the bride's retinue and members of the audience. Deprived of his vision, Arno had to determine which of the women in line was Sabine by touching each of their hands in turn. When he reached my "bride," who had inserted herself midway into that line, he felt her hand, trying to discern if it belonged to Sabine. Hoping to encourage Arno to move on after lingering, she gave him a nudge, which the poor fellow mistakenly took as a signal from Sabine, whom he had dated for years. When he removed his blindfold, Arno stood stunned. He glanced over at Sabine, who was frowning, and immediately dropped to his knees in front of her, hands joined in supplication, pleading forgiveness. A howl of merriment rang through the hall. Feigning irritation, Sabine stamped her foot and folded her arms in a gesture of disgust. A barely perceptible smile crossed her lips.

The students had dressed me in a red satin jacket with a pattern of circular white medallions and dark slacks reminiscent of those worn by scholars during the late Qing dynasty. My bride wore a close-fitting red vest, embroidered with silk, the sleeves of which stopped halfway down her upper arm. A light-colored skirt accentuated her dark brown hair (pulled back in a bun), light makeup, and red lipstick. She looked all the world like a porcelain doll. Her lithe figure and delicate features, distinguishing characteristics of women from Jiangsu province, evoked the elegant and cultured heroine of the novel *Dream of the Red Chamber*, Lin Dai-yu. To embellish our costumes and to set the scene, our students supplied us with a long twine rope and a red veil.

In imperial China, the practice of arranged marriages often meant that a bride and groom would not see each other before the wedding, and to heighten suspense for all involved, the bride remained veiled during the procession and the ceremony. My students tied a rope around her waist and gave the other end to me. I led her onto the stage in a manner that reinforced traditional patriarchy and attitudes towards women in an age of polygamous marriage. Once the other rituals were completed, I hesitantly removed her veil. Feigning great pleasure at scoring such a fetching wife, I turned so that she could jump on my back, as instructed, and I circumambulated the room comically to the amusement of the audience before exiting stage right. That ritual—which the students chose—represented a husband taking a wife away from her parent's home.

I left Shanghai in August to arrange a small apartment in Denver and to get ready for the three courses that I'd be taking each quarter—and the two that I'd be teaching. I used the Internet to find rental listings and an old road atlas to locate them. I had hoped to live within walking distance of campus, but despite assurances from the apartment building manager about the unit's proximity to the university, I eventually had to get a car. With student loan funds, I purchased the white Civic wagon in which Tony drove us to the emergency room two years later. By the time I picked Savannah up from the airport in mid–December, I had grown a full beard and shaved my head. Thus, rendered unrecognizable, I inadvertently frightened her in the airport lobby. When she saw me approach from the corner of her eye, she jumped back and let out a short shriek.

On the way home from the airport, we stopped at Fazoli's, an Italian-American chain restaurant on the route home. On that snowy mid–December evening, the waitress brought us two cups of ice water and placed them on the wooden bistro table where we had seated ourselves among a profusion of restaurant logos. "Why would anyone serve water with ice cubes on such a cold night?" Savannah wondered aloud, wrapped in a red down jacket, dark hair falling over her shoulders. When the waitress returned to take our order, she requested a cup of hot green tea, ubiquitous in China, but the restaurant carried only flavored teas: orange, peppermint, cinnamon, blueberry. Savannah opted instead for a hot chocolate, and while the pasta was nut-free, it wasn't especially flavorsome. On many occasions in later years, Savannah would dine with me at restaurants chosen more for ingredients not listed on the menu than the appeal of the food they served.

During the winter break, we jumped into the Honda with one backpack each and left the Mile High City for Las Vegas. Our route took us over the Rocky Mountains, across the Continental Divide, and through the Martian-like landscapes of southern Utah. Our first night on the backroads, which we had chosen to avoid interstate highways, the sky was clear. A full moon blanketed the road ahead in soft white light. We marveled at the immensity of the landscape and the shining silver stream to our right that sounded softly through the closed windows of the Honda. The shadowy outlines of the canyons rose on our left like ghosts against the darkness. I wondered what would happen if our car, which we had bought used and had not owned for long, broke down in the "middle of nowhere." We didn't carry a cell phone, at that time a luxury item, and did not have an American Automobile Association membership for emergencies. Luckily, I had thought to have the Civic serviced for a road trip, and we arrived at our destinations without incident.

A few days before Christmas, the scrubby slopes of the Nevada desert gave way to a sea of lights as we neared Las Vegas. Since it was the off-season, we took a heavily discounted room at the Hilton, which was promoting "Star Trek: The Experience," a multimillion-dollar themed installation. Imagine, Starfleet officers on the bridge of the *USS Enterprise*, and Klingons, Borgs, Ferengi serving Cardassian ale and "blood" wine at Quark's Bar. After two nights of marveling at the kitschiness of it all, we checked out and made our way to the Little White Wedding Chapel, where we got married, in our car, for $35. As we entered the Drive-Thru Tunnel of Vows, its ceiling painted sky blue with naked cherubim floating through misty clouds, a good-humored priest dressed in black stepped out. Through the driver's side window, he had us recite wedding vows. When the time came to exchange rings, we looked at each other, and turned to the priest: "Sorry, we don't have any." A veteran of the unusual wedding scene in Vegas, the gentleman barely batted an eye, and then pronounced us man and wife. We drove out of the wedding chapel to a bed and breakfast near the Grand Canyon. The following day, we passed through Santa Fe, and stopped in Taos for the night, before heading back to Colorado. To avoid tree nuts on that trip, we stopped at local grocery stores for bread and sliced meat to make sandwiches.

Not long after returning to Denver, Savannah enrolled in a master's program at University of Colorado and won an internship in a teaching program at Stanley British Primary School. We moved into a small one-bedroom apartment belonging to the school on the former site of Lowry Air Force Base. Because that small two-story apartment building originally housed visiting officers who ate on base, it did not have a kitchen. So, we bought an electric wok and rice cooker to prepare simple meals, and we washed dishes in the bathroom sink. A pair of old handcuffs, locked around the bedroom doorknob, proved a source of humorous speculation for us and for our occasional guests. During that time, I used to grab a Philly steak sandwich at a local haunt where my friend Wesley, who knew about my food allergy, tended the grill, and we found a fabulous family-owned Korean restaurant, called Myeongdong, where Savannah enjoyed a variety of dishes, while I predictably stuck with *bulgogi* (sliced beef), white rice, and *kimchi*.

The following summer, we moved to California so that I could teach a couple of classes for the Summer English Language Studies program at UC Berkeley. In the small house that we rented for three months, I typed up an application for a Fulbright graduate teaching assistantship in Turkey on an ancient typewriter (belonging to the homeowner), which made each letter higher, then lower, than the one preceding it. To my great surprise, I won that fellowship, presumably because of the experience teaching in South Korea and China and the argument I made about wanting to learn more about the histories, cultures, and literatures of the Middle East. In 2001, I took a leave of absence from the University of Denver for one year and later that summer stayed at Dad's house in Virginia to await the visa paperwork. Excited at the prospect of a new international adventure, we anticipated having time to visit friends and family in Richmond before flying to Turkey. It was there, late one night, that I mistakenly ate the pecan cookie that put me on a ventilator.

-◊-

The anaphylactic episode that begins Chapter One leaves off at the moment I lost consciousness. You will recall that I got out of the Honda and fell to my knees in front of the emergency room doors, thus bypassing admission and triage. By the time I was seen by medical staff, just 35 minutes or so had elapsed since swallowing the pecans—and I was confused, blue, and on the verge of passing out. Had the police car that followed us part of the way to the hospital pulled us over, and a few more minutes elapsed, I might not have made it to Turkey, finished graduate school, found a teaching position, or penned any books. The world would have been no poorer for my absence, but I like to believe that two subsequent decades of teaching and writing has made some contribution to the common weal.

After I was admitted to the hospital, Tony phoned Mom to let her know what had happened. It was the middle of the night. "Nikki, this is Tony. I don't want you to worry, but Mark's in the emergency room. Nikki, don't cry." He also comforted Savannah, who was frightened, still in her pajamas, and in tears. In Shanghai, she had once performed the Heimlich maneuver on me when I choked on a large multivitamin. For some inexplicable reason, that frightening event endeared me to her, and thereafter Savannah has felt some obligation to look after me.

On this occasion, I fell into systemic anaphylaxis after losing consciousness and was administered epinephrine at intervals of five to ten minutes for bronchospasm, hypotension (abnormally low blood pressure), and angioedema (swelling that becomes threatening when it causes the throat or tongue to block airways). The two most common errors associated with mortality in severe anaphylaxis are delays in administration of epinephrine and intubation. Because of the swelling of my tongue and throat, doctors sedated me so that a flexible plastic tube could be inserted into my windpipe to maintain an open pathway for air. Imagine trying to insert such a pipe down the throat of someone already struggling to breathe and in shock. Sedation, which also erased much of my memory of this experience, proved wise, and once intubated, attendant physicians hooked me up to a respirator that kept me alive for 24 hours while my body endured rebound anaphylaxis.

The primary cause of death from anaphylaxis is airway compromise or cardiovascular collapse—and, as we have seen, fatal anaphylactic reactions are more common in patients with asthma.[3] People suffering severe anaphylactic reactions, especially those rapid in onset, are at greater risk of rebound (biphasic) anaphylaxis. Dr. Torrisi, the pulmonologist on call, stabilized my condition, and transferred me to the intensive care unit, where I awoke the next day, in hospital bed number seven, hooked to IV drips and medical machines—just like when I was a kid. The breathing tube had been removed shortly before I was summoned back to consciousness, and my throat, trachea, and chest were sore. At least, a tracheostomy had not been necessary. I was fortunate to survive given the severity of this allergic response and the fact that endotracheal intubation is a high-risk procedure in ICUs and sometimes results in mortality. Too much oxygen poisons the sacs that pass air into the red blood cells, worsening the condition of the lungs, but too little of it impairs the brain and kidneys. The possibility of brain damage is also far higher following complications in the ICU where the physiological instability of the patient compounds such risks (unlike with stable patients intubated in the operating room for surgical procedures).[4]

When I awoke from sedation, I opened my eyes to find Dr. Torrisi leaning over me. I remember his long face, strong chin, salt and pepper hair, and warm smile. Looking at me with clinical curiosity, he asked somewhat humorously, "You're the Fulbright scholar?" Confused but responding in the affirmative seemed to suggest to the good doctor that I had escaped the worst of the dangers of intubation due to his first-rate care. My mother, who arrived at the hospital shortly after Tony's call, must have told Dr. Torrisi that we were moving to the Middle East for a year. I wonder what he thought about that plan, after saving my life?

-◊-

The experience of losing consciousness in the emergency room, being intubated in the ICU, and waking up to a doctor leaning over me to check for brain damage from lack of oxygen, radically changed my understanding of the severity of the food allergy. When it came time to eat in the hospital before discharge, the paper slip used to order that meal read "NO NUTS!!!" in capital letters. To stay alive going forward, following that injunction would remain vital. Although aware of the reputation of the Fulbright program, Mom was hardly thrilled with the prospect of our leaving for Turkey in a few weeks—but the job market for full-time English professors was abysmal (and is even worse now), and I thought that moving to Ankara to teach for a year would improve my chances of landing a tenure-track teaching position after graduation. During my short convalescence in the intensive care unit, I remarked to a nurse that I had never experienced such a devastating allergic reaction. Her reply remains seared into my mind: "they tend to get worse each time." While researching this book, I learned that is not *always* true, but the trajectory of my allergic reactions to tree nuts has been that they generally worsen. For that reason, I now live as if the next time will be the last.

Living the Food-Allergic Life

After release from Chippenham Medical Center, at 32 years of age, I finally accepted the reality of my condition. From then onward, I strove for total avoidance of tree nuts, wore medical alert jewelry, and carried epinephrine anywhere there was a possibility of eating. Making those lifestyle adjustments seemed easy compared to dealing with the paralyzing fear of food that I experienced, which, though somewhat attenuated, persists to this day. Suddenly, even when I could be almost 100 percent certain that a meal did not contain a trace of tree nuts, I began to avoid eating. I also considered declining the Fulbright award and had plenty of opportunities to do so, since it would be late September 2001 before the visa paperwork was completed—just after the terrorist attacks that made many Americans reassess the safety of airline travel, as well as the wisdom of living and working in the Middle East. Declining that award would have hurt my chances on the job market, but more importantly it would have meant allowing food allergies to circumscribe my activities and to define my identity.

We left for Turkey three weeks after the World Trade Center towers came down, and I would have to find safe meals for at least nine months in a country known as the "hazelnut capital of the world."[5] Before getting on that plane, I had learned that nut-filled pastries were popular in Turkey and that traditional Ottoman fare often contained tree nuts (frequently pureed in sauces, making them difficult to identify on sight).

Unlike South Korea and China, where tree nuts in traditional dishes are rarer, Turkey presented a new series of challenges—including how to deal with the post-traumatic stress of surviving a series of severe allergic reactions to food. In my view, the psychological dimensions of living with potentially fatal food allergies are among the most overlooked aspects of that disease process.

-◊-

Before moving on, permit me to note several alarming statistics regarding the rising prevalence of food allergies. They increased by 50 percent between 1997 and 2011 in children globally, and the prevalence of peanut or tree nut allergy more than tripled in American children between 1997 and 2008.[6] Approximately 40 percent of children with food allergies have experienced a severe allergic reaction such as anaphylaxis.[7] Around 30 percent of children with food allergies are allergic to more than one food—and approximately 170 foods have been reported to cause reactions.[8] Allergies to milk, egg, wheat, and soy sometimes resolve in childhood, but children seem to be outgrowing some of these allergies more slowly than in previous decades, with many children remaining allergic beyond the age of five. Childhood hospitalizations for food allergy also tripled from the late 1990s to the mid–2000s.[9] In addition to the difficulties of ensuring safe meals at school, children with food allergies are twice as likely to be bullied compared with children who do not have a medical condition.

Just eight major food allergens—milk, egg, peanut, tree nut, wheat, soy, fish and crustacean shellfish—are responsible for the most serious food allergies, though concerns are emerging regarding sesame as well.[10] Allergies to peanuts, tree nuts, fish and shellfish generally persist throughout life. In the following pages, we review the promise of the early introduction of allergens (in place of simple avoidance), oral desensitization regimes in a medical setting, and even traditional Chinese medicine in treating severely allergic individuals and improving their quality of life. For the time being, advances in food labeling in the United States and around the world are essential to helping people avoid allergens, though the dangers of cross-contact during food harvesting, transportation, storage, manufacturing, and processing are real. Most people will understand that experiencing anaphylaxis, struggling to breathe, and blacking out a few minutes after mistakenly consuming trace amounts of a forbidden food can be terrifying, especially when rebounds occur for hours, or even days, afterward. Given the centrality of food to sustaining health, and to culture and society more generally, grappling with the fear of food after surviving anaphylaxis presents a series of vexing challenges highlighted in the next chapter.

CHAPTER THREE

All Fears Great and Small
-or-
Scared Witless
and Afraid to Show it

"...but death is the most terrible of things; for it is the boundary; and beyond that nothing appears to the dead man either good or bad."
　　—Aristotle, *The Nicomachean Ethics* (350 BCE)

"...who would [burdens] bear,
To grunt and sweat under a weary life,
But that the dread of something after death,
The undiscover'd country from whose bourn
No traveller returns, puzzles the will,
And makes us rather bear those ills we have
Than fly to others that we know not of?"
　　—William Shakespeare, *Hamlet* (1599–1601)

-◊-

According to influential psychologist Abraham Maslow, food, water, and shelter are among our most basic physiological needs, and without them we struggle to access higher levels of motivation and meaning in life.[1] In addition to our innate biological need for the nutrients and energy that come from food, most of us recognize that food is also socially sustaining. Among early human beings the quest for food encouraged the formation of cooperative foraging groups. A trial-and-error process, presumably informed by an intuitive fear that new foods could prove harmful, tempered a desire among early humans to try unknown foods to determine their edibility. An inborn aversion to bitter foods protected the body from dangerous toxins, while a bias towards sweetness and the texture of fattiness facilitated quick energy

58

boosts.[2] The taste buds on our tongues discern sweetness, saltiness, bitterness, sourness, and savoriness, and the odors drawn through the nose, together with the sight of food, helped to measure its capacity to satisfy the hunger instinct.

We are omnivores, all-devouring beings capable of consuming meat and plant foods, and we possess a unique evolutionary adaptation that kept us from depleting the environment by encouraging the discovery of new food sources in other regions. Social groups classified foods into those that were edible and non-edible and used culture to formulate rules about how and when to consume those deemed acceptable. The successful selection of stable, edible food choices by social groups sustained human populations for generations.[3] Some cultures suffused food classifications with dietary prohibitions related to moral or religious beliefs and designated certain foods as pure, clean, and safe—or, conversely, as impure, polluted, and dangerous.[4] Over time, culture shaped tastes for certain flavors and created cuisines that drove strategies for food acquisition, organized food production, and influenced interactions with other cultures and the environment.

Although we must "eat to live," the need for food is much more than a biological imperative. Food helps to define personal and group identity, molds our habits, influences our health, and engages our hands and minds in its procurement, preparation, and consumption. Because social groups make food choices part of moral and ideological agendas, preparing and sharing food serves as a primary form of in-group sociability. Through a process of socialization and enculturation, people acquire food preferences, and the flavors, smells, and appearance of food remind us of who we ate with before, and in what place.[5] Everywhere around the world, friends, family, and groups share meals to reinforce social ties, forge communities, and foster loyalties and obligations.[6] Several times a day, meals provide an opportunity to affirm relationships in accordance with cultural norms of etiquette. When someone transgresses those rules, as sometimes happens inadvertently to people with severe food allergies who adopt strategies to keep safe, such as refusing dishes or not attending meals, it could signal rejection of hospitality or even of a particular cultural or social group.

Although how we eat, what we eat, when we eat, and with whom we eat varies from place to place, from culture to culture, from group to group, and from era to era, food provides a marker of heritage and identity and binds us together in important ways. People find conviviality around food and tend to eat more when together than when alone. Food prepared in the home may be conceived as a gift, a silent act of benevolence, that ties families together and carries a tacit expectation of balanced reciprocity (in which food-allergic people may not be able to fully participate). In other words, food is about much more than individual and group survival, it is integral to many social and cultural systems. Even our increasingly busy modern lifestyles have not displaced the centrality of cooking and eating to our social lives.

Yet, for those of us living with food allergies, an invitation to someone's home for breakfast, lunch, or dinner poses challenges, due to the need for strict avoidance of staple food ingredients such as milk, wheat, soy, nuts, fish, and shellfish. Restaurants make meals transactional by stating prices and offering sustenance outside of regular mealtime hours, but they are also sites of danger for food-allergic people regardless of the style of the restaurant (fast-food, ethnic, fusion, family style, and so on). "Bring-a-dish" events and holiday celebrations can generate alarm in people with food-induced anaphylaxis due to the threat of undisclosed ingredients and the possibility of cross-contamination. In other words, the integration of food with so many aspects of culture and society means that allergic individuals must maintain vigilance to avoid allergens, while simultaneously negotiating social situations involving food in ways that do not offend hosts or unnecessarily draw attention to themselves. Such people must also grapple with fears that arise from repeated exposure to food antigens, fears reinforced by negative experiences (i.e., anaphylaxis) after eating.

For someone like myself, a survivor of several anaphylactic reactions, a buffet held at work to reward employees, to celebrate a group accomplishment, or to build community becomes instead a source of worry. While others may relish the prospect of a free meal, I approach the buffet event with apprehension. Imagine a large conference room with a wooden stage decorated for a festive occasion. After the director, a tall woman dressed in a beige pantsuit, her brown hair pulled back in a ponytail, delivers cheerful opening remarks, she invites everyone to queue up at the buffet tables set up at the back of the room. The caterers, dressed in white, stand in front of steaming food trays with folded paper labels placed neatly in front of them identifying the dishes: stir-fried rice, barbeque ribs, tortellini, chicken scones, pasta with pesto sauce, samosas, multigrain bread, and a double chocolate cheesecake for dessert.

After grabbing napkins, utensils, and a plate, I scan the buffet table for dishes unlikely to contain tree nuts. In such situations, my preference leans towards food prepared in the simplest way: a piece of grilled chicken with salt and pepper, a baked potato, corn on the cob, a boiled egg. At this event, the buffet table is not allergy friendly—nor is the side table set up and staffed by employees who brought dishes to share. For many reasons, I often prefer not to publicly identify myself as someone with life-threatening food allergies. At the catered buffet table, the stir-fried rice, barbeque, pesto sauce, multigrain bread, samosas, and chocolate cheesecake potentially contain nuts as an ingredient. As I survey the employee offerings, a friendly and clearly famished person to my right—speaking loudly enough for others to overhear (perhaps the chef)—suggests amiably: "You should really try some of Kimberly's potato salad; she brings it every year, and everyone raves about it!" A non-allergic person, who doesn't really like potato salad, might smile, and reply, "thank you for the recommendation," and put a bit on her plate for the sake of politeness.

Knowing that tree nuts sometimes feature in potato salad recipes, I nod thoughtfully at the suggestion but must pass over the dish discretely. Such behavior might be interpreted by others as rude, or at least peculiar, especially if Kimberly is within earshot. Alternately, I could hold up the line to ask Kimberly if she used tree nuts in her recipe, but since trace amounts can trigger anaphylaxis, there's still the possibility of cross-contact. Perhaps she ground walnuts for a cake and then used the same spatula to stir the potato salad? Maybe her cutting board wasn't cleaned thoroughly after chopping almonds and still contained residual proteins when she sliced potatoes on it? Do I inquire further, and reveal my medical condition, or keep moving? From my vantage point, neither is a good option. Either one might make me seem awkward, picky, eccentric, when I'm simply trying to avoid anaphylaxis.

Likewise, the decision to skip events where known food allergens are present in the environment can leave one open to accusations of snobbery and a lack of "team spirit," but deciding not to eat at such events is fraught with its own difficulties. Consider the following imaginative reconstruction drawn from actual situations. The boss hires the most popular local Vietnamese restaurant, The Saigon, to cater this year's Labor Day picnic. Because peanuts and tree nuts feature in many dishes on their menu, I know that trying to find a safe meal at the picnic will be nearly impossible, and ultimately not worth the risk. Plain white rice could have been one safe option, but the rice and noodle dishes, sauces, and marinades might contain finely chopped ingredients that could prove deadly. Rather than risk it, I eat something before the party and attend to socialize with friends and colleagues. It's easier to escape unwanted attention when there's no single time for everyone to sit down and eat together. But should the boss make a presentation first, and then invite everyone to the repast, then I'm the only one who does not queue for food, and who sits at a picnic table without a plate. To make matters worse, I'm quite thin.

"You're not hungry?" asks Joan, a pleasant woman with blonde hair wearing a green dress and stylish burgundy glasses.

"I'm fine—and hope that you enjoy your meal!"

"Why don't you get something to eat?" asks John from accounting.

"Oh, I'll get something later. What did you think of the speech?" I ask trying to change the subject and to steer attention away from myself. If I respond by explaining that I have an extreme food allergy, that information usually elicits further scrutiny and prompts stories of others they knew—or heard about—with similar allergies, usually of varying severities. John might ask, "What are you allergic to?"

"Tree nuts."

"What happens if you eat them?" queries Joan.

"I could die within thirty minutes without medical care." Silence.

"I read in the paper about a teenager who died after mistakenly eating peanuts at summer camp," offers Glen, the 6'5" former high school football player in operations management. "It must suck having that kind of allergy. I love to eat!"

A similar scene played out recently at an end-of-the-year union meeting at the college where I teach. Because so many faculty and staff members had already left town for the summer, the event was rescheduled from Pizza Land, a local Italian-American restaurant where I sometimes eat, to a lovely log home outside of town owned by one of our Executive Board members. Leah, a gracious and hospitable woman, and her husband Rick took the initiative to order food for their guests from their favorite barbeque house in Binghamton about 70 miles away. Leah, a retired faculty member, made sure that I took a soft drink when I arrived. When lunch was served after some official business, about ten to twelve folks found seats around a patio table on their deck overlooking the town of Oneonta below. "You're not eating, Mark!" Leah exclaimed, obviously disappointed considering the length of their trip to the barbeque restaurant.

From prior experience, I knew to regard barbeque sauces as potentially dangerous. Years earlier, again at my father's house, I bit into a chicken leg, and my mouth immediately started burning. I spit the chicken out, opened the refrigerator, read the sauce label, and, sure enough, almonds were among the last ingredients listed. Although that allergic reaction was mild, because I did not swallow the chicken, I avoid barbeque sauces unless I can review the ingredients. Not wanting to explain that history to the work group assembled to share a meal, I simply replied, "Thank you, Leah. I'm good." In truth, I would have eaten something if they'd ordered from Pizza Land, but I wasn't starving.

"No wonder you're so skinny," someone at the table remarked with a mouth full of food.

"It's unhealthy not to eat," offered Rick. "My mother died from not eating."

-◊-

My father's "almond experiment," and the mother of my friend Mark who treated his asthmatic episodes as panic attacks, exemplify a once widely held view that food allergies and asthma were conditions with symptom sets rooted in anxiety disorders such as hypochondria. Since food allergies are an "invisible" illness, unless one discloses them or has a reaction in front of you, dealing with them in social situations can be perplexing. Fortunately, heightened public awareness in recent decades means that food allergies are taken more seriously now—especially in children and teens. Some states, including Massachusetts and New York, have eliminated all peanut products from public school classrooms.[7] In Canada, the Province of Ontario implemented Sabrina's Law in 2006 to train staff members and to develop emergency plans for students with anaphylactic allergies following the tragic death of 13-year-old Sabrina Shannon from cross-contamination in a school cafeteria.[8] Sabrina's Law ushered in a new era of protection for food-allergic children at risk of anaphylaxis, but it required mandatory disclosure of health status.

By keeping environments free of foods that could cause anaphylaxis, Ontario schools sought to accommodate at risk children, but the requirement to disclose led to *felt* (anticipated) and *enacted* (experienced) social stigmas. The unintended consequences of the well-meaning protective policies in Sabrina's Law created tension between children's physical safety and their social well-being. While appreciating the need to keep children with severe allergies away from food triggers in school, I also recognize that the social consequences of being stigmatized are easily overlooked. An individual's social identity, in this case as a severely allergic person, permits others to determine how that person fits into their world. When a perceiver's expectations about a person's health, which are largely reflective of social norms in a particular time and place, are not met, it creates a negative social construct that stigmatizes the ill person as abnormal or inferior.[9]

Enacted or experienced social stigma involves labeling, stereotyping, exclusion, discrimination, and loss of status. If an allergic person identifies with such labeling, it becomes internalized and subsequently shapes life chances (employment, housing, overall welfare). Those with infectious diseases, mental health issues, alcoholism, physical disabilities, and "deviant" or non-normative bodies often report health-related stigmas.[10] For people with invisible health conditions, such as anaphylaxis and epilepsy, the decision to disclose comes at a cost. One study found that epileptics attempting to cope with the negative social implications of their condition either concealed their health status to avoid social unacceptability, downplayed their condition unless it was necessary to disclose, or advertised it to educate others and to avoid negative judgment.[11]

Severely food-allergic people must avoid food antigens, eliminate them from the home, and reduce contact with public and private spaces where they might be present. Because of that necessity, they often end up limiting social contact as a means of protecting their physical safety and well-being. A growing body of medical literature makes clear that allergic people feel socially isolated from peers and family members, anticipate anxiety in public spaces and in social settings, and experience heightened levels of fear in their everyday lives. In the next chapter, we turn to the role that parents and caregivers play in keeping their children safe, meal after meal, by teaching them to read food labels, minimizing their exposure to unsafe settings, and making sure that they carry epinephrine. Sabrina's mother understands "social isolation from anaphylaxis can be lonely" because "much of the world, particularly family and social events, revolves around food."[12] She describes Sabrina as a "social butterfly" whose allergies relegated her to a lunch table away from her classmates and excluded her "from activities and birthday parties."[13]

Many young people with food allergies experience bullying at school, especially in grades seven to ten when perpetrators are more likely to touch, wave, and throw allergens—*or even to intentionally contaminate food*. Such bullying erodes quality of life for allergic

children and increases the distress of their parents. Only recently have researchers begun more methodically exploring the psychosocial consequences of living with life-threatening food allergies. Social stigma and exclusion can worsen existing health issues, with stress being the primary mechanism for that intensification. Such outcomes tend to be magnified in young people at psychologically and socially formative times in their lives. For this reason, anaphylactic youth are more likely to ignore food labels and to enter unsafe environments without epinephrine injectors to fit in with peer groups.[14] Although anaphylactic adults encounter peers less frequently who bully in the same manner as kids in middle school, many of the same factors leading to social stigma apply.

I hesitated to disclose my food allergy during the multi-day "on campus" job interviews that I had after graduating from the University of Denver—despite having to take several meals at restaurants with potential colleagues during the interview process—for fear of being negatively stigmatized. After all, I thought, who wants to hire someone for an appointment leading to lifelong tenure when that person could "kick off" after eating dinner? While my experience may not be typical, I have never received an offer for a fulltime teaching position after disclosing the food allergy, usually out of concern about meal safety at restaurants chosen by the hiring committee. In a profession that puts emphasis on collegiality, finding someone who gets along well with other members of a department can be more important than a candidate's credentials. For that reason, I've found that it often "doesn't pay" to disclose in such situations, even if that omission puts my life at risk.

-◊-

The gourmet food revolution of the 1980s brought best-selling books, popular magazines, television shows featuring celebrity chefs, and entire television networks dedicated to food. The type of journalism that Anthony Bourdain innovated in *A Cook's Tour* (2001) contributed to the growth of food tourism, and the international focus of his television show *No Reservations* (2005) highlighted the political, social, and cultural relevance of food by illuminating the web of symbols, images, practices, and beliefs that form around cuisine.[15] Bourdain's work demonstrated the way in which food provides a prism through which to explore the art, history, and cultural traditions of people around the world—and it showed how shared meals reinforce mutual bonds and unite those who participate in them.

Living the Food-Allergic Life

Nonetheless, foreign cuisines, ethnic foods, and culinary tourism present challenges to people with food-induced anaphylaxis that are hard, though not impossible, to overcome. I recently heard about a friend of a colleague who packs an entire suitcase of kosher cereal in order not to transgress religious food prohibitions, and she eats that cereal every day, for every meal, while traveling. I never went to such extremes to avoid tree nuts, and such measures would make little sense on extended stays of months or years, but I often pack a few nonperishable lightweight foods whenever feasible. It makes good sense, particularly for people with multiple food allergies, to bring along a supply of safe nonperishable foods (egg replacer, sesame-free bread, nut- and soy-free cereals, gluten-free pastas) when traveling.

Negotiating the cultural and social dimensions of food as a severely allergic person often proves as difficult as practicing strict avoidance during international travel, particularly in countries where one cannot read or speak the language. No human being can escape the natural conditions that make eating, drinking, and socializing vital to a healthy life. Meals bring people together, but they can also divide us when one cannot participate or is excluded from them—and the hesitation to share food in foreign countries when it is offered may be misinterpreted. People living with severe food allergies may also miss out on pleasurable experiences associated with food that create positive memories that allow people to relive the past in various ways. The smell of food evokes powerful memories, sensations, and emotions: the gingerbread cakes wafting from the oven in grandmother's house at Christmas, granddad's homemade baked ziti, the beans and franks stirred over an open campfire during summer vacation. By contrast, in anaphylactic individuals, food memories can take on a more sinister cast and produce emotional reactions associated with pain and suffering.

Allergic children often carry associations of food with anaphylaxis into adulthood. The secondary psychological complications (comorbidity) experienced by a seven-year-old boy with a peanut allergy highlights the potential for negative associations with food, as well as a propensity for profound anxiety, difficulty getting along with peers, and family disruption. This child, whom researchers called Billy, exhibited behaviors indicative of obsessive-compulsive disorder. He frequently washed his hands, reported regular thoughts of being contaminated by peanuts, and asked his mother for reassurances about safety from peanut exposure multiple times per day. Billy refused to eat food that his mother had prepared, if she had consumed peanuts earlier in the day, or if she

used ingredients from sealed jars positioned near cans of peanuts.[16] He stopped eating lunch at school and avoided school personnel, in case they'd been in contact with peanut products.

Allergic reactions to food can be traumatic for adults, as well. After suffering a major reaction at work and being hospitalized, Kate Hufnagel was diagnosed with allergies to peanuts, tree nuts, lentils, sunflower, sesame, and artichokes at the age of 38; she now carries epinephrine and restaurant allergy cards and always wears a medical ID. An adult food allergy diagnosis, especially one revealed through anaphylaxis, "tends to give way to a variety of emotions, including fear, anxiety and concern about social isolation."[17]

High levels of anxiety in asthmatic children are also well-documented, including the "panic" that many experience during the onset of an asthma attack.[18] Children with food allergies may also develop anxiety disorders and should be taught to distinguish the physiological symptoms of hyperventilation from an allergic reaction. Helping children and teens to discern the difference between physical symptoms of anxiety and the first signs of anaphylaxis that they mimic can reduce the unnecessary use of medications, such as epinephrine, in response to anxiety, which is important since epinephrine worsens panic attacks by speeding the heart rate and increasing nervousness. Not being able to breathe during an asthma attack—and the sudden onset of life-threatening anaphylaxis—are traumatic experiences, and it makes sense that some residual anxiety would surround them.

The trauma resulting from the rapid onset of anaphylaxis can also produce high levels of vigilance following each episode, which may develop into eating disorders. Conversely, prolonged periods between allergic episodes tend to lower anxiety and relax vigilance—and by failing to exercise sufficient caution, new accidental exposures may occur, which subsequently strengthen apprehension about eating.[19] Careful reading of food labels, always keeping epinephrine on hand, using safety protocols for food preparation, and curtailing activities that involve eating in uncontrolled environments can help children and young adults to cope, whereas a lack of understanding, an unwillingness to accommodate, and even open hostility from family members, friends, neighbors, and school personnel hinder the successful management of food allergies. Most incidents of food-induced anaphylaxis occur outside the household (often at restaurants, school, and work), and the greatest number of fatalities from food-induced anaphylaxis take place away from home.[20]

Living the Food-Allergic Life

We generally associate post-traumatic stress disorder (PTSD) with surviving military combat or exposure to war zones; natural disasters, serious accidents, physical or sexual assault, life-threatening injury; or the sudden violent or unexpected death of someone close to us. However, a recent study investigating the psychological mechanisms involved in the development of PTSD symptoms after anaphylactic shock found that the trauma of this distressing abnormal event alters an allergic person's relationship to the environment and can lead to the development of symptoms including hypervigilance, anxiety, and depression.[21] Such individuals may feel that their sense of safety has been violated, or that they are unable to terminate a potential threat, which in turn generates high levels of uncertainty that impact the ways they cope, especially after repeated exposures.

Distressing, unpredictable, and potentially life-threatening medical emergencies necessitate changes in a patient's relationship to the environment. Post-anaphylaxis, some people become preoccupied with dangers in their immediate environment and conduct ritual checking, which does little to abate uncertainty about whether food eaten will provoke a reaction. Instead of enjoying a restaurant meal or a dinner party with friends, anaphylactic people live with a fear of food, which is part of a complex emotional and behavioral response that is difficult for people without food allergies to understand. One study of anaphylactic shock survivors found that more than 90 percent reported feeling extremely fearful about what happened to them during anaphylaxis. A large proportion of the survey group experienced tingling, burning lips, swollen mouths and tongues, and difficulty breathing. Sixty percent found blisters or large red wheals on their body, and 23 percent fell into unconsciousness. About 12 percent of those surveyed met the diagnostic criteria for PTSD.[22] A more recent survey of Korean adults with life-threatening food allergies found a "remarkably high prevalence of PTSD and associated psychological distresses" in survivors of anaphylaxis that "have a direct effect on the quality of life."[23]

The more severe the post-anaphylactic PTSD symptoms, the more often patients employed problem-focused, emotion-focused, and avoidance-focused coping strategies. Medical intervention for people who experience anaphylaxis tends to focus on relieving the physical symptoms of the disease to save lives, but too little attention is given to the subsequent psychological challenges of living with food allergies. I'm unsure if my repeated, increasingly severe, exposures to tree nuts have resulted in post-anaphylactic PTSD or are simply indicative of a conditioned response in which associations are formed between food and life-threatening illness, but I employ many of the coping strategies outlined above—and I struggle at times with unfounded fears of food.

-◊-

Today, most physicians and medical researchers acknowledge that severe food allergies can result in emotional problems, including, but not limited to, irritability, nervousness, depression, despondency, and envy of one's untroubled peers. When a food-allergic person distrusts the safety of various foods to an extreme degree and excessively limits their diets, those behaviors indicate an overactive protective response to a frightening event (or series of them), in this case anaphylaxis. Anxiety resulting from eating something one wrongly believes contains an allergen can turn into a panic attack, which mimics the symptoms of a food allergy (hyperventilation, difficulty breathing, rapid heart rate, dizziness, nausea, faintness). Such episodes of terror without an obvious *external* cause (i.e., the lack of allergens in the environment to trigger anaphylaxis) represent fear responses that become maladaptive.

Sandra Schwartz experienced a serious allergic reaction in August 2005 that left her too frightened to eat foods known to be safe. A couple of days after suffering anaphylaxis to shrimp, she went on a camping trip in remote Northern Ontario when she suddenly felt unable to breathe. Worried, her boyfriend drove her as quickly as possible to the next town, but once in the hospital parking lot, Sandra realized that she wasn't experiencing an allergic reaction, but a panic attack. "I just sat crying in the car," she remembered; it was then she "realized that there's a real psychological element" to her condition.[24] Even after that epiphany, she only felt safe eating cereal and pasta. Three months after the camping trip, she had lost twenty pounds. Lauren Alexander, diagnosed with a tree nut allergy as a baby, lived a normal life until she ate a nut-laced salad dressing in a restaurant, which afterward plunged her into a state of alarm in which she felt continually surrounded by foods that could kill her.[25] In the most extreme cases, food-allergic individuals become afraid to eat altogether and slip into anorexia, experience panic at the slightest sign of an allergic reaction, and withdraw from society to avoid further exposures.[26]

Such responses may strike many readers as irrational, but as Scott Sicherer, a pediatric allergy specialist at Mount Sinai School of Medicine, observes, "If I stood next to you, pulled out a gun and held it at your head, you're going to shake, you're going to sweat, and you're going to fear for your life, because you know that gun could hurt you. So if you've been hurt by food, that type of fear can become a huge part of your existence."[27] Schwartz confesses that, years after anaphylaxis, she still experiences anxiety every time she goes out to eat, tries a new food at home, or shares a meal at a friend's place, but she asserts, "I'm not going to let that stop me. I just have to live life."[28] Parents and caregivers may suffer from similar fears about the safety of their food-allergic children.

Everyone, without exception, experiences fear. This universal human emotion, evoked by challenges in the environment perceived as threatening to one's survival or wellbeing, means that we fear separation from a safe base, places lacking an escape route to safety (buses, trains, and airplanes), and closed spaces such as elevators. We fear predatory animals, domestic pets (particularly dogs), and a variety of smaller often harmless creeping and crawling insects and reptiles. Some fear social rejection; criticism by others; targeting by aggressive or violent people; injury, illness, or surgical procedures; and, of course, death.[29] Fear provides a means of coping with adverse and unexpected situations by activating the nervous system to provide metabolic resources for forceful action, and by mobilizing defense behavior (avoidance or "fight or flight").

Fear makes the brain hyperalert, raises the heart rate and blood pressure, and accelerates breathing. It speeds the flow of blood around the body, causes pupils and bronchi to dilate, facilitates the flow of glucose to skeletal muscles, and slows organs not vital to survival.[30] Fear is rooted in biological evolution to provide a way to manage dangers by alerting us to potential threats to our integrity or existence. In primitive organisms, the fear response tends to be highly reflexive, such as the recoiling of a worm pecked by a hungry bird.[31] The small black and white jumping spider, determined to weave a web between the table and the patio chairs, exhibits a reflexive fear response and instinctively recoils with every thump of my finger. Were that spider to jump on my arm and move toward my face, before I could consciously weigh the negligible threat such a tiny creature posed, I might inadvertently kill it by reflexively brushing it off.

While evolution primes our responses to fear, fears can also be learned (or conditioned). Predators in the wild provide clues to their presence in the faint sounds they make, and the odors that exude from their bodies, which their prey learn to interpret as life-threatening

70

signals that elicit fear and defense responses.[32] When an association is formed between two stimuli (such as a sound or smell with danger), it can be recalled later to activate the state of fear more quickly. Seven-year-old Billy provides an example of people with anaphylactic food allergies who exhibit a conditioned fear response to food. Yet, this natural critical avoidance response is not invariably beneficial. The expectation based on past experience, that avoidance produces safety, is easily confirmed and provides a basis for a cluster of behavior patterns that we might informally call "playing it safe."[33] When fear develops in a way that is out of proportion to the objective danger of a situation, an otherwise healthy fear response slips into the realm of phobia (the irrational fear of specific situations or events) and anxiety disorder (which affects up to 25 percent of the population).[34]

Phobias and anxieties interfere with the ability to successfully manage many of life's challenges; they limit choices and generally have a detrimental effect on well-being. Anxiety-disordered people tend to overestimate the probability of life-threatening events and to exaggerate their negative consequences. To qualify as an anxiety disorder, fear, anxiety, and avoidance must be persistent and either cause significant personal distress or impair daily functioning.[35] Consider the individual with an intense and irrational fear of flying who nevertheless must travel internationally for work, which causes her great anxiety. After retirement, however, that person never needs to fly again, and thereafter would no longer suffer the harmful consequences of that fear of flying. Unfortunately for those of us with severe allergies, who develop phobias and anxieties around food, there is no way to avoid eating.

-◊-

In hindsight, I realize that just a few weeks after surviving anaphylaxis in Richmond, I was unprepared for the fear of food that accompanied me to Ankara, Turkey. Aside from the stress of moving to a new country, of teaching new courses, of attempting to learn a new language, like everyone else, I had to eat several times a day. The terrorist attack on September 11, 2001, had delayed our visa documents, and my three communication courses in the International Relations department at Middle East Technical University were already underway when we arrived. Mercifully, someone from the Fulbright Commission had arranged faculty housing on campus for us, which meant that we would not have to find our own apartment in the sprawling city.

Living the Food-Allergic Life

Before that last dance with anaphylaxis, I had looked forward to living abroad again; to learning more about Turkish culture, history, literature, and art; and to acquiring new perspectives from people with different backgrounds and worldviews. Upon arrival, I found myself with just a Turkish-English dictionary to look up words for different types of nuts, a phrasebook with essential entries for medical care, and few Turkish friends who could help me negotiate restaurants and read food labels. We shopped at the small convenience store on campus, but soon figured out how to take the *dolmus* or minibus from school to the grocery store, about 20 minutes away, where we could buy fresh meats and vegetables, pasta, rice, and other staple foods to cook at home.

Although homecooked meals didn't often generate trepidation during our stay, there were times when concerns about the ingredients in packaged foods arose. Had I mistakenly eaten that chocolate chip cookie at my Dad's one or two years earlier, I would have reconsidered Turkey as a Fulbright destination. On the other hand, having that anaphylactic episode so exquisitely fresh provided the hypervigilance required to survive for two semesters. Were it otherwise, repeating the risky eating habits that I foolishly practiced in East Asia might have resulted in death. Although sometimes irrational, the fear of food that I developed in Ankara had a positive impact on my ability to avoid meals containing even trace amounts of tree nuts. Yet, "playing it safe" resulted in the formation of a cluster of avoidance behaviors and coping mechanisms that are unhealthful, and it curtailed the traveling we did in Turkey and other countries in the region and limited our social interactions.

Handsomely situated at an ancient crossroads connecting Europe and Asia, the Anatolian peninsula has sustained human communities since prehistoric times. The ancient Assyrians and Hittites colonized it, the Greeks settled its western coast, and the Persians conquered it during the sixth century BCE. From the second century BCE onward, western and central Anatolia came under Roman rule, and by the fourth and fifth centuries Turkey had become part of the Christian Byzantine Empire. Turkmen from Central Asia gradually encroached on Byzantine holdings until a Turkish tribal leader named Osman (from whose name the term "Ottoman" is derived) spread Islam and extended his rule over the entirety of Anatolia. When Ottoman forces led by the 21-year-old Sultan Mehmed sacked Constantinople (modern-day Istanbul) in 1453, they vanquished the Byzantine Empire and created an imperial central government that would endure until the early twentieth century.

Chapter Three. All Fears Great and Small

At the pinnacle of its power, under the rule of Suleiman the Magnificent, the Ottoman Empire stretched northward into Eastern Europe, southward through the Levant and into Egypt and Arabia, and westward across north Africa and into southern Spain. As the Industrial Revolution bolstered the political, economic, and military power of Western Europe during the nineteenth century, the Ottoman Empire fell into decline. During the Great War (1914–1918), a navel raid against Russian ports on the Black Sea coast caused the Allies (Britain, France, and Russia) to declare war on the Ottomans. At the Battle of Gallipoli, not far from the ruins of Troy, a fabled city celebrated in the *Iliad* (c. 8th century BCE), a dashing young general named Mustafa Kemal Atatürk defended the coast from invasion. Following Ottoman capitulation, he led the Turkish National Movement, founded the modern Republic of Turkey, and served as the nation's first President from 1923 until his death in 1938. During that time, Atatürk secularized the country, opened thousands of new schools, introduced a Latin-based alphabet, and granted Turkish women unprecedented civil and political rights.

Atatürk may have made Ankara the political capital of Turkey, but Istanbul remains the nation's cultural center. The Bosphorus Strait divides Istanbul into eastern and western districts and connects the Black Sea to the Sea of Marmara, and it provides access to trading routes throughout the Mediterranean. Noteworthy landmarks in Istanbul include the Byzantine Hippodrome built in 203 CE, the Hagia Sophia (Church of Holy Wisdom) that boasted the largest dome in the world for almost 900 years, and the giant Basilica Cistern built in 532 by the emperor Justinian. Ankara, where the Fulbright Commission placed me, may not rival Istanbul as an historical and cultural epicenter, but it became the nation's political capital in 1923 following the war for independence against proxies of the Allies.

Located deep in the traditional heartland of Anatolia, Ankara is an ancient urban center founded between two rivers on the eastern edge of a great plateau. Positioned amid fertile steppe land and forested hills, summers in Ankara are hot and dry, and winters are cold with occasional snow. Part of the traditional Hittite homeland referenced in the Hebrew Bible, Alexander the Great conquered the city in 333 BCE. Ankara passed into control of the Roman Empire around 25 BCE, and it remained an important center of commerce under Byzantine rule until the seventh century. Orhan Gazi, son of Osman Gazi, captured the city in 1356, and the Ottoman timber houses near Ankara Castle remain one of the most interesting parts of a city that includes ruins of a Roman bath, the Temple of Augustus and Roma, and many impressive mosques. The remarkable Museum of Anatolian Civilizations is also housed in Ankara. From this brief overview, it's easy to understand why Turkey seemed a place uniquely suited to gaining a better understanding of the histories and cultures of the Near East.

-◊-

Unfortunately, my difficulties with food started on our first day in Turkey. We woke up in the neat, small, one bedroom flat reserved for us on campus and made our way to the Fulbright office downtown by hailing a taxi at the front gate of the university. It surprised me to discover two guards dressed in green fatigues and armed with assault rifles at each side of the gate checking identification papers and waving vehicles onto campus. In the guardhouse, students and visitors on foot checked in before proceeding to class and other appointments. On the way to the Fulbright office, we got our first glimpse of the bustling city: bright three- to four-story concrete and glass buildings, restaurant tables and chairs neatly arranged under patio awnings, street vendors with carts on bicycle wheels under colorful umbrellas selling all kinds of food from corn-on-the-cob to sesame buns (*simit*) and roasted nuts.

After several attempts, our taxi driver located the Fulbright Commission in Ankara's affluent embassy district by following the address listed in Turkish on a business card—our sole connection to the office's whereabouts. We walked a block or so down one of the walled streets around the embassies and entered the white stone building that our driver pointed toward before letting us out. When we entered, we were greeted by the secretary and shortly thereafter by the assistant director of the Fulbright office, an elegant middle-aged woman with dark hair and bright, intelligent eyes. After briefing me on the Turkish Fulbright program, lecture and travel opportunities, and events planned throughout the year, Ms. Solak offered us red tea served in small hourglass-shaped glasses with silver spoons for stirring in cubes of sugar. She also brought out a circular plate featuring varieties of Turkish Delight (*lokum*), a confection made by mixing chopped dates, pistachios, hazelnuts, or walnuts with honey and molasses.

Having just survived anaphylaxis, the sight of those confections filled me with foreboding. Savannah took a piece from the plate for the sake of politeness, but I declined by explaining that I had a severe food allergy to tree nuts. It took a few moments for the full impact of that explanation to sink in, but when it did, Ms. Solak looked at me thoughtfully and remarked: "You had better be really careful this year; nuts are a common ingredient in Ottoman cuisine." That fact meant bakeries would be off limits and eating in most restaurants would be impossible due to the possibility of miscommunication, cross-contamination, and hidden allergens in sauces and marinades. Turkey also had a lower incidence of food allergies than the United States, which meant hospitals would be less accustomed to treating food-induced anaphylaxis, and restaurant workers wouldn't always understand the need for complete avoidance. On the positive side, the commission would pay for Turkish lessons, though I had to commute downtown five days a week to take that opportunity. As I taught and read for the dissertation, Savannah researched John Dewey's role in the development of secular primary and secondary education in Turkey for her master's thesis.

McDonald's, the only restaurant where I ate during that nine months, had conveniently opened a branch on campus, not far from foreign faculty housing. It was a small-time affair in a building that looked more like a cottage than a restaurant, and it had just enough room for four cashiers and a prep area. I availed myself of it frequently and enjoyed eating outside on sunny days on the benches and picnic tables that surrounded it. Many stray dogs and cats prowled around the forested areas of campus. Some of those unfortunate critters suffered abuse at the hands of children and unsympathetic adults, and their bodies betrayed evidence of that mistreatment. One famished feline, a tabby, leered at me menacingly one day as I was about to take a bite of a Big Mac. Amused, I began to tease it, but that mangy little creature grabbed the entire sandwich out of my hand. Surprised and a little bit alarmed by the cat's vehemence, I recognized a soul hungrier and feistier than my own—and watched it devour my sandwich.

I took a packed lunch and grabbed a *dolmus* downtown for Turkish lessons during the fall semester. Most of my fellow students were from Central Asian and African nations, and they studied at various universities in Ankara, often on Turkish government scholarships. I enjoyed meeting them and learning Turkish, but between the *dolmus* operators, who wouldn't depart until most seats were full, and the teaching and research obligations, by the end of the semester those lessons no longer seemed manageable. Having to walk by so many street vendors and their carts of freshly roasting nuts, spewing allergens into the air, wasn't fun either. As I passed one nut cart after another, I held my breath or pulled the collar up to cover my nose. In researching this book, I learned that airborne food allergens (in powdery form or from cooking) rarely induce anaphylactic reactions, though it does happen.[36]

The most surprising challenge that year came from post-anaphylactic fears of meals prepared at home with ingredients purchased at the supermarket or from the little store on campus. Some forms those fears took remain embarrassing to recount, but I share them in the hope that they prove useful to others. I took "test runs" to the nearest hospital with 24-hour emergency care and a ventilator (about 13 miles or so from campus) and determined that the trip took 20 to 25 minutes one-way in the middle of the night and about 35 to 40 minutes during the day, if it wasn't morning or afternoon rush hour. None of those figures included the time it took to leave the apartment and hail a taxi. Such travel times meant that any accidental ingestion of nuts in packaged or pre-prepared foods would necessitate the use of one—perhaps two—EpiPen's along the way. After the episode in Richmond, I knew the onset of shock would make it difficult to communicate in English (let alone Turkish) during an emergency. I wore the medical alert necklace that Mom bought for me after the last hospitalization, but the message imprinted on the back "anaphylaxis to tree nuts" was written in English.

Out of an abundance of caution, I consulted with hospital staff, alerted them to the possibility of food-induced anaphylaxis and asked them to make that condition part of my medical file in the event of an emergency. On more than one occasion, when some part of a carefully prepared home cooked meal made my tongue or mouth tingle in a way suggestive of the presence of an allergen, we would grab a taxi, rush to the hospital, and sit in the waiting room anticipating the symptoms of anaphylaxis. After a couple of hours, if signs of food allergy did not appear, we'd return home. On one such occasion, I recall sitting with my back to the wall watching people come through the emergency room doors. After we had been there for some time, a hospital staff member asked us, in English, to check in if we needed help. I explained my food allergy to her, and the lingering fears of another dance with anaphylaxis, and she allowed us to stay until we felt comfortable leaving.

Foods such as bananas, spinach, red or black peppers, and other spices sometimes made my mouth itch suggestively, but they elicited no allergic symptoms. Even so, those itching sensations created anxiety that triggered panic attacks, which reinforced the perception of the onset of anaphylaxis. Even when eating carefully prepared meals, I sometimes became hostage to fear. The tightness in the chest, the shortness of breath or sensations of suffocating, the accelerated heart rate, the trembling or shaking that characterized panic attacks reinforced the feeling that anaphylaxis would follow. Not being able to read food labels well (even with a dictionary) added to my concerns about ingredients in foods that were otherwise safe for me, such as canned tomato sauces.

My determination to stay alive in Turkey also meant avoiding working lunches with colleagues and meals at friends' houses. Perhaps most disappointingly, we curtailed our travels around Turkey, though we availed ourselves of two-to-three-day bus trips to places such as Cappadocia, Istanbul, and Mount Ararat. On those occasions, Savannah, who bore all this post-anaphylactic anxiety with great patience, made me a thick crust pizza that I would eat for breakfast, lunch, and dinner—even when it became soggy after a day or so. I felt awkward eating homemade pizza when everyone else stopped for restaurant fare—but it was safe.

During the winter break, we spent a few days in Italy, where we saw our friend Giuseppe, then an assistant professor of law, whom we had met at UC Berkeley. A small, sweet man with a warm smile and hazel eyes, Giuseppe invited us to his parents' home in the countryside of northern Italy. His mother accommodated me with homemade ravioli and his father with delicious sausages made from scratch. Except for the two days that we spent with Giuseppe, I survived on cheese pizza, which may seem somewhat "nuts" to those who travel overseas and enjoy trying local cuisines. My confidence in cheese pizza as a means of survival was deeply shaken when a hunt for lunch in a small café in Sienna turned up square sheets of white pizza, with a big, fat walnut on each slice. Having foregone sauces, stuffed shells, baked goods, and desserts (including gelato) in Italy, this blow left me feeling vulnerable.

-◊-

After returning to Turkey, Savannah left to visit her parents in China for a month. I fended for myself by keeping the diet simple, buying foods labeled for international sale with ingredients listed in English, cooking raw meats and vegetables, and sticking with familiar brands of pasta and rice. Even in the United States, food labels are sometimes inaccurate and manufacturing mistakes happen, recipes change, and cross-contact with allergens occur. In fact, undeclared allergens remain the number one reason for American food recalls.[37] More than twenty years after last having anaphylaxis, the reading and re-reading of labels, often multiple times, if the list of ingredients is long and printed in a small font, remains a daily ritual. Those who regularly peruse food labels understand how difficult it can be to remain mindful while noting every ingredient. Consider, for example, this comparatively brief list on a package of white tortillas:

> Ingredients: whole wheat flour, water, enriched bleached flour (wheat flour, malted barley flour, niacin, reduced iron, thiamine mononitrate, riboflavin, folic acid), soybean oil and fully hydrogenated cottonseed oil, leavening (sodium bicarbonate, sodium aluminum sulfate, calcium sulfate, monocalcium phosphate, corn starch), contains 2% or less of each of the following: sugar, salt, palm oil, hydrogenated soybean oil, fumaric acid, sorbic acid, sodium stearoyl lactylate, sodium sulfite, cellulose gum, maltodextrin, carrageenan. Contains: Wheat

Or this label from a package of instant noodles:

> Ingredients: wheat flour, palm oil, potato starch, modified potato starch, salt, beef seasoning (yeast extract, beef bone stock, beef extract, liquid corn syrup, beef tallow), monosodium glutamate, dehydrated vegetables (green onion, mushroom, carrot), red pepper, sugar, soy sauce powder (hydrolyzed soy protein and corn gluten, maltodextrin, salt), soy bean paste powder (soybean, maltodextrin, salt), soy bean paste powder (soybean, maltodextrin, salt), black pepper, garlic, red pepper seed oil, potassium carbonate, oleoresin capsicum, oleoresin paprika, onion, corn, ginger, sodium carbonate, disodium inosinate, disodium guanylate, sodium metaphospate, sodium tripolyphosphate, sodium phosphate, T-BHQ, sodium pyrophosphate, riboflavin color.
>
> Contains wheat and soy. Manufactured in a facility that also processes eggs, milk, fish and shellfish.

If your attention lapsed even briefly while reading these lists, you will understand why making reading labels part of a daily mindfulness practice is important, for when attention falters or one starts to skim labels, it creates an opportunity for accidental exposure.

-◊-

Among the lost opportunities in Turkey to food allergy: traveling with other Fulbrighters to Antalya, a city on the Turquoise Coast of the Mediterranean known for its blue waters, to celebrate the end of the academic year. Food in Turkey varies significantly by region (fish and greens in the Black Sea region, wild herbs and mutton in the high steppes, peppers and spices in the southeast, and cheese and yogurt in the northeast). Due to Anatolia's long history as a nexus of trade between Asia and Europe, and as the center of the Ottoman Empire,

Turkish cuisine fuses many culinary traditions: seafood and olives from the Mediterranean coasts; spices from the Far East; nuts and dried fruits from the Middle East and the Levant; rice, grains, legumes, and cured meats from central Anatolia.[38] Negotiating that rich culinary landscape proved a perilous proposition for me—just as Ms. Solak at the Fulbright office had suggested it might.

Nuts—most conspicuously walnuts, almonds, hazelnuts, pistachios, and chestnuts—lurked in unexpected places: meatballs, cooking oils (hazelnut and walnut), pasta dishes, pancake omelets (*kaygana*), stuffed vegetables (*dolma*), chicken soup (*tavuk corbasi*), and most conspicuously in all manner of desserts (*halva*, *baklava*, Turkish Delight). Even kababs could contain ground walnuts mixed with spices, and because of such seasoning mixes, I also avoided *doner*, a popular roasted meat cooked on a vertical rotisserie and sliced to order. As tempting as it was to try, and it was on more than one occasion, my goal was to stay alive and learn as much about Turkey as possible.

I have passed on meals that were probably safe in the United States, and still do, but my biggest food regret in Turkey was not joining a meal with a colleague and his family. Psychologically, I was not prepared for it. Bill and Afifi lived nearby in faculty housing, a cluster of small bungalow-style buildings containing four one-to-two-bedroom apartments with kitchenettes and living areas separated by bar-like countertops. A visiting scholar from University of Canterbury in New Zealand with a specialty in political science, Bill had short grey hair, a medium build, a gentle manner, and the slight stoop of a scholar dedicated to writing. His exuberant Lebanese wife, Afifi, and their three exceptionally bright children, shared a flat surrounded by cypress and juniper trees on the northern edge of campus. Behind them, a wooded hill where we occasionally hiked. Bill and his family traveled with us on a couple of sponsored trips for visiting faculty members—and they knew the challenges that I faced eating in Turkey. Afifi, perhaps not fully cognizant of the severity of anaphylactic reactions, invited us over for a traditional Lebanese meal—*sans* nuts.

We accepted because I thought that I could eat without fear, but even before dinner was served, I became filled with great uneasiness. Despite assurances from Bill that "there wasn't a nut within a mile of the food tonight," I knew that nuts were part of their daily diet and could be found in their kitchen cabinets. So, I worked on a computer problem with the boys while everyone else ate. Not only did I miss this opportunity, Afifi must have been disappointed after she spent the better part of a day preparing that meal. Although I was not able to articulate the fears and anxieties that assailed me that year, I hope that they may have encountered other people with anaphylactic food allergies in the intervening twenty years and have forgiven me.

Although fear and hypervigilance diminished my experience in Turkey, I worked with some amazing students and managed to successfully finish that teaching assignment. I returned to Denver "skinny as a rail," according to my department chair, but "alive and kicking." We moved to an apartment on Warren Avenue across from the university, where I could finally walk to campus. Nevertheless, I continued to experience high levels of apprehension around food and increasing social awkwardness in situations where food was served.

-◊-

Some behaviors that I developed post-shock represent avoidance strategies that emerged in response to negative stimuli or "punishment" (i.e., anaphylaxis). When an activity followed by punishment is abandoned, new avoidance behaviors develop passively. Conversely, behaviors form actively after learning that a particular action or activity enables the avoidance of punishment.[39] Passive avoidance suppresses existing behavior, while in active avoidance new behavior is acquired.[40] It's difficult to extinguish conditioned responses in food-allergic people because it's impossible to ingest a trigger allergen without the unconditioned response (allergic reaction), which would lower fear levels. Any attempt to eliminate the avoidance response (that is, not eating when food cannot be deemed safe) might result in a loss of protective behavior and encourage risky eating. So, if one can't expose a patient to the stimuli she fears by having her ingest allergens without a severe allergic reaction (something only possible if current efforts at allergen-specific immunotherapy proves successful)—and you can't punish the avoidance response, as one might with behavioral treatments for phobias and other neurotic conditions—then it becomes very difficult to eliminate or to positively transform avoidance strategies in people with deadly food allergies.

Over the past several years, I've noticed a tendency to practice passive avoidance behaviors by not eating anywhere where tree nuts are likely to lurk, and I no longer travel internationally much. I have made exceptions since last experiencing anaphylaxis to build a career in a highly competitive discipline, but at considerable personal expense. After graduating from the University of Denver, for instance,

Chapter Three. All Fears Great and Small

I taught fulltime in the English department at Drake University in Des Moines, Iowa. During my campus interview, a two-day affair involving five-to-six meals at local restaurants, I did not disclose my food allergy. When I met Provost Troyer, a hardworking Midwesterner with a Mennonite background, he seemed interested in my international teaching experience. Before I taught the first class that fall, the Provost invited me to his office to explain that the prior semester he and the President had attempted to set up an exchange program to encourage Drake graduates to teach in China. The first seven participants were facing challenges living and teaching in a provincial Chinese city—and the dean coordinating the exchange had recently departed. Given my experience in China, he asked me if I could help put the new program on surer footing.

At that time, the President and Provost were receiving regular calls from concerned parents of graduate teachers in Hebei Province, and given the gravity of the situation, they invited Savannah to join the team as an assistant director. We dove in, and the Chinese Cultural Exchange Program (CCEP)—which planned community events, coordinated faculty exchanges, and recruited graduate teachers—was established. We traveled to China twice during the fall semester to address the problems of alumni teachers. While it was an honor to have worked for CCEP, the banquets with college and university administrators in China, and the travel to other parts of the country to find new exchange partners, proved a challenge. With a native Chinese speaker accompanying me, I could choose restaurants and make food choices that were reasonably safe, but the highly social nature of Chinese banquet culture repeatedly put me at risk.

One of the ways I handled trepidation about eating in China was to simply resign myself to the fact that I could die during those trips. The final chapter of this book addresses the power of that kind of surrender, and the focus on the here-now that it engenders, but I was keenly aware of the risks that I was taking during those trips to the Far East. It's difficult to explain the nuances of the Chinese banquet model of dining, but it is crucial to building relationships and to doing business in the Middle Kingdom. These examples of the avoidance behaviors that follow helped me to survive potentially dangerous encounters with tree nuts, but they engendered instances of social awkwardness that could have been misinterpreted as cultural insensitivity.

Returning to China as an assistant professor and director of a small China program brought opportunities to learn about that country from a different perspective. Rather than teaching writing and literature courses, here was an opportunity to develop faculty and student exchange programs. The frenetic pace of development in China during the mid–2000s defies imagination. Construction cranes hung over every street corner, and entire city blocks could disappear, then be rebuilt, almost overnight. It surprised me to find a huge twin tower in the middle of the Fudan campus made of glass, steel, and a stone façade. It seemed better suited to the business district in downtown Shanghai, for most of the other buildings on campus were only a few stories in height. Initially, the chance to return to China in a different capacity seemed wonderous, since it provided a window on the break-neck pace of change in the country. Mindful of limited budgets, we always traveled modestly. Finding universities and colleges that would agree to offer our graduates English language teaching positions, and to host our scholars and researchers, meant traversing that enormous country on demanding time schedules. While the regional cuisines of China gave cause for concern, the banquets remained the biggest obstacle to staying safe.

Within a couple of years, the joy of those trips turned to dismay at the prospect of busy eight-to-ten-day schedules involving multiple stops around China. The fact that these journeys always took place during the semesters, while I had courses running, made them more difficult. Having Savannah along alleviated some worry about finding meals when we were alone, but such occasions were relatively rare. Unlike their American counterparts, Chinese colleges and universities shut down completely during summer and winter breaks, so we had no choice but to travel during the semester. The flight from Des Moines to Beijing or Shanghai took around 24 hours, including layovers. We learned to stay overnight after arriving, rather than catching connecting flights to Guangzhou in the south or Sichuan in the southwest. Although CCEP hosted a few Chinese scholars on long-term exchanges, our main goal was locating institutions of higher learning where recent graduates could teach English language for one or two semesters. We made sure that such positions included round-trip airfare, housing (typically a private studio apartment near campus), a salary that constituted a fair living wage for the area, and holiday breaks for travel.

On a typical trip, we would take a train from Beijing to Hebei province in the morning (a three-hour trip one-way at the time), visit our graduates, meet with administrators, and give presentations to students interested in studying abroad at Drake. Always gracious hosts, Chinese administrators frequently invited us to lunch and dinner banquets, public activities of considerable social import. Because Chinese society tends to be hierarchical, seniority and rank were clearly established during group meals. The president of the university (or other senior official) sat at the head of a large, usually circular, banquet table, while those occupying lesser ranks would position themselves on either side, in descending order. The closer one sat to the "boss," the more important they became in the eyes of others. Elaborate rituals of deferential social tiering played out in which lower-ranked employees poured drinks for the higher-ups, selected the best dishes for them, and listened attentively as they spoke.

Rather than the buffet arrangements many Americans are familiar with (where one selects from items set out with their own dedicated serving spoons or forks), Chinese banquets are typically held in the private backrooms of popular local restaurants. In the center of each table usually sat a large round Lazy Susan (rotating tray) on which were placed an astonishing number of dishes, ordered in advance and served one-by-one in a staggered fashion over one-to-three hours. One always sat in the assigned place designated by the host, and initially just water and a couple of snack dishes were placed on the table: nuts, sliced fruit, dried vegetables. The reader may think that it would be easy enough just to avoid the nuts by not touching them, but etiquette allows everyone at the table to use their chopsticks to select items from dishes, which always raised the specter of cross-contamination. Imagine someone uses her chopsticks to take an almond from a plate on the Lazy Susan, eats it, then uses the same chopsticks to select a piece of chicken from a dish that might have otherwise been safe for me.

On more than one occasion, Savannah snatched dishes with nuts from the table before everyone sat down and returned them to the kitchen with as little ado as possible. Well-meaning hosts, who encouraged me to try special dishes, proved challenging—as did the constant toasts with beer, wine, and *baijiu* (a strong rice liquor), which loosened people up and fostered trust and bonding. For fear of causing offense unintentionally, I turned down food as politely as possible, usually by explaining that food allergies limited my diet or by claiming to be full. Because I didn't want to refuse toasts as well, I tended to drink too much at banquets, but it would have been hard to make any deals in China had I passed on those too. Negotiating breakfast buffets at international hotels was a bit easier, since fewer people joined us and dedicated serving utensils for dishes were standard. Most mornings, I got by on a boiled egg, bowl of white rice, and green tea.

Living the Food-Allergic Life

One morning in Chengde, a small city in Hebei Province north of Beijing where the Qing dynasty Kangxi emperor kept a grand imperial summer residence, a college staff member encouraged me to try the local milk. When I saw that the small white can had pictures of almond blossoms on it, I declined with some difficulty and silently marveled at the unexpected dangers lurking at every meal on each trip. Because tree nuts grew in abundance in this region, they featured prominently in local cuisine, a fact that heightened vigilance. Our travels to Sichuan province also proved troublesome, since the hot red pepper sauces the region is known for might be nut-free, but they burned the tongue suggestively and raised concern. No longer dogged by the terror that assailed me in Turkey, traveling with CCEP still meant facing the fear of eating in a foreign country. Because the onset of anaphylaxis can be delayed for hours—and even days—the "game" of waiting for symptoms to emerge after a fear-creating meal remained disconcerting. For that reason, I took advantage of the opportunity to grab a quick meal at American fast food restaurants when possible. The easily identifiable ingredients of a hamburger (a white bun, a meat patty, something resembling cheese, ketchup, mustard, and onions), potato fries, and a soft drink decreased worry.

I said a prayer of thanks each time we returned home safely from trips scheduled so tightly that we often slept in a different Chinese city every night, and met new students, faculty, and administrators every day. We ran CCEP from 2004 to 2007, and I'm thankful for the opportunity to build that program, which at the time of writing was still in operation using the model that we set up. It proved gratifying to work with college graduates who benefited personally and professionally from teaching in China, but the difficulties that regular business travel to China presented meant somewhat reluctantly leaving Des Moines to teach for a comprehensive college in the State University of New York system.

-◊-

Following the rigors of travel with CCEP, I passed on other opportunities to teach and travel overseas for ten or so years. During the summer of 2013, I agreed to offer two English language courses on the campus of Hankuk University of Foreign Studies in Seoul for two weeks. That assignment meant taking a break from researching *Palace of Ashes* (2015), but I wanted to get a better sense of how South Korea had changed since the late 1990s (it was more developed, more outward

84

looking, and more vibrant). By this time, 14 years had elapsed since the last anaphylactic reaction in Richmond, and I thought that I could better handle eating in a foreign country, especially one with familiar foods. Though I didn't expect a repeat of the extreme fear that held me in its clutches in Turkey, it returned with a vengeance on the flight across the Pacific Ocean.

I must have been nervous because I left for Albany International Airport around 5 a.m. without eating. At that time of morning, during the summer, it's a beautiful one-and-a-half-hour drive up Interstate 88 through the foothills of the Catskill Mountains. The rising sun bathed the scenery in warm yellows and golds. I arrived an hour or so before the short flight from Albany to JFK in New York City, and during the layover in the airport lounge ate one of the pasta noodle burritos that Savannah had prepared. That left one more for the 14-hour leg from JKF to Incheon International Airport. After being herded into the Boeing 747 and finding my window seat, it wasn't long after takeoff that a snack of mixed nuts was served. The two women to my right both enjoyed their tree nuts, but their pungent odor signaled danger to me. My mind began wandering into fanciful scenarios of contamination from oily fingers and of an allergic reaction from inhaling nut particles in the stale air of the plane.[41] With the aircraft flying over the Arctic for hours, my mind played all kinds of tricks on me as I peered down into the vast and beautiful expanse of ice and snow below. The in-flight navigation system playing on the large screen in the aisle between the seats made clear that there would be nowhere for an emergency landing should I slip into anaphylaxis. I declined the meal of "chicken or fish" when dinner was served, and made the mistake of not eating anything, even the food Savannah made, during the duration of that transcontinental flight.

Cruising at 30,000 feet, the cabin air in the plane is always dry, and in economy class, flight attendants never seem to serve enough water. Before long, I became hungry, weak, and dehydrated. My body began to smell sour, so much so that on the one-hour car ride from Incheon to Seoul, I cracked the passenger window of the car and apologized to the program representative who picked me up, explaining to her that I was sick. Having lived in the country before, I knew that Koreans thought that foreigners smelled anyway, and well understood that my present condition affirmed those cultural assumptions. She kindly offered to take me out for dinner after that long flight, but fearful of what restaurant might be chosen, perhaps something fancy, which posed a greater risk, I asked to be dropped at the hotel in the Hwigyeong Dong neighborhood of Seoul instead. A long driveway led to the hotel, a small four-story building situated within walking distance of classrooms and offices on campus.

I made another error in deciding not to finish the remaining burrito at the hotel. It had butter and cheese on it, and after about 30 hours of traveling with me unrefrigerated, it made a soggy and unappealing option for a meal. Since it was so close to dark, I fell asleep exhausted and hungry on the twin bed of the small second-story room. By the next morning, I hadn't eaten anything for almost 40 hours and was much the worse for it. Like a car driven too long without refueling, my body began to run out of energy. Being so thin, I had few reserves to keep going. In extreme cases, when the body depletes its fat reserves, it begins breaking down protein in muscle tissue. In my case, the beginning of that process resulted in the weakness and stomach cramps associated with decreased metabolism. Within a couple of days, my teaching duties would begin, and in this compromised state, I began to wonder if I could meet those responsibilities. Fortuitously, before departing, I had arranged to meet my old friend Dr. Park from Masan for lunch the day after my arrival.

After I left South Korea for China in 1998, Dr. Park retired from Kyungnam University and had been working in Seoul. A short, friendly man, usually dressed in slacks, a blazer, and a button-down dress shirt, Dr. Park's dark eyes flashed with good humor, the deep furrows running down his cheeks rose when he smiled. Because I had not eaten in so long, he found me in a pitiful state. To cure my ills, he proposed rice soup from the Lotte World department store downtown. I managed to walk to his large black sedan, but rather than sitting in the passenger seat, I huddled in a fetal position in the back seat, occasionally moaning. Too weakened to enter Lotte World, I remained in the massive parking garage, while Dr. Park located a restaurant serving rice soup. He bought a large container of it, which I lived on for two days as I recovered my strength. Even though I was starving, at first it was hard to eat much. Gradually, I began to feel better and hunted out other food possibilities for the next 12 days.

Eating three meals a day would mean finding 36 safe meals, but if I reduced that number to two, that meant just 24. I could do it! Save for a trip the following week to a music store, and a couple of sightseeing excursions with Dr. Park, I limited my activity to the ten or twenty blocks around the university and the hotel. One of the staff members at the front desk told me that a local McDonald's delivered, and I also found a Burger King about ten minutes away by foot. Those two establishments provided a welcome opportunity to eat with less fear. Near the hotel, I discovered a family-owned Korean restaurant with patio dining where you could watch the world go by on the streets of Seoul. I stuck to two dishes during my stay: *galbitang* (a clear beef rib soup with radish, onions, and a few glass noodles) and beef cooked on the table with garlic and served with a bowl of rice and a side of *kimchi*. The *galbitang* proved a powerful restorative as the teaching began. How fortunate to find that restaurant and to have remembered a bit of Korean, but I was glad to return home after teaching.

The apprehension that I had experienced from the flight to Seoul onward rivaled that in Turkey, when I scouted out hospitals and made occasional runs to the emergency room believing that I had eaten something nutty by mistake. Although such levels of unhealthy anxiety cannot be sustained for long, that fear response helped me to remain alive in Turkey. On the other hand, the food fears in South Korea were largely unnecessary, given the low incidence of tree nuts in Korean food. With the benefit of hindsight, it would have been prudent to book a hotel with a kitchenette, but then again, the host school arranged those accommodations, and my stay was short. I try not to let food allergies limit my actions, or to become too problematic for other people. But, as the next chapter demonstrates, it's not just those with food-induced anaphylaxis who suffer the consequences of severe allergies—it's often the people around them, too.

CHAPTER FOUR

Upon Others, Our Lives Depend
-or-
Those Who Help and Those Who Harm

"God has made us so that we must be mutually dependent. [...] The most proudly independent man depends on those around him for their insensible influence on his character—his life."
—Elizabeth Gaskell, *North and South* (1854)

-◊-

Families coping with the diagnosis of any chronic disease face challenges to which individual and collective responses vary considerably. Parents of children with food-induced anaphylaxis will struggle to sustain elimination and avoidance diets, especially in large families, in ways that do not discriminate against allergic children or subject them to resentment by siblings deprived of a favorite food. Meal preparers must constantly screen ingredients while balancing the taste preferences of everyone in the home. Because keeping allergic children out of harm's way requires everyone to learn new behaviors (reviewing ingredients of every food product entering the home, carrying first aid kits, educating allergic individuals, and learning to administer injections and provide cardiopulmonary resuscitation), household members may develop feelings of hostility, experience embarrassment in public, or express difficulty in accepting the severity of food allergies.[1]

Unfortunately, some children grow up with people who lack sufficient concern to remove allergens from the home environment or simply do not want to give up beloved foods and snacks on their account. Tree nuts, for example, were always present in my father's house, and my stepmother relied on me to read food labels when I had concerns about ingredients, rather than parsing long lists on packaging herself. The more severe the allergy, and the greater the burden of care, the more likely children will become the object of deep-seated antipathy or ridicule, even though such attitudes often prove hurtful to children who are quick to internalize such mindsets. Billy's mother reported feeling annoyed that she and her husband could no longer enjoy peanuts in their own home. She mocked Billy when he refused to kiss her after she had eaten peanuts—and when he declined dinner, if she had eaten peanuts prior to cooking—despite his pediatrician's warning that minute peanut particles on her mouth or hands could induce an allergic response.[2] Such attitudes have been implicated in increased morbidity among children with asthma and food allergies.

As young people with food allergies reach school age, vigilant parents will worry about allergens in school cafeterias, about kids swapping foods during lunchtime, and about food-bullying.[3] In decades past, parents, teachers, and administrators dealt with such apprehensions individually, meaning they usually lacked a uniform institutional strategy to protect these children. A recent study with more than 4,500 participants concluded that 64 percent of allergic children experienced reactions while in daycare or in school, most of them unexpected or accidental.[4] Twenty-five percent of participants reported having their first food-induced allergic reaction in an educational setting after ingesting a previously unrecognized antigen.[5] Most allergy specialists emphasize that the best way to manage extreme food allergies is to practice absolute avoidance, but that strategy leaves parents and caretakers in a conundrum given the ubiquitousness of some allergens, such as milk and egg, in the diets of most children.[6] Outright bans on certain foods from educational environments unduly impose upon families whose children do not have food allergies—and they can lead to teasing and to bullying of the allergic "culprit."[7]

Because food allergy awareness and management in school has now become more common, parents of children with a confirmed IgE-mediated food allergy should compile and submit a food-allergy action plan. Such a plan typically contains medical information that outlines the cause of allergic reactions, lists medicines and emergency contacts (including doctors), provides access to prescribed epinephrine and medicine protocols, and includes a blueprint for securing immediate medical care in a facility prepared to handle anaphylaxis.[8] Teaching and support staff must learn when to notify families whose children share classrooms with allergic peers, and they should also receive training in reading food labels and recognizing anaphylactic reactions and be given easy access to epinephrine auto-injectors. Even "allergy-free" cafeterias and classrooms cannot operate safely without trained staff who can identify common allergens, prevent their introduction into foods, and spot potentially life-threatening situations.[9]

Sometimes, the discovery of allergies to food and other triggers (medications, insect stings, latex, strenuous exercise) comes only after an unexpected reaction results in a trip to the emergency room and a new diagnosis. In *Feeding Eden* (2012), Susan Weissman recalls that her son Eden, who had been diagnosed with a milk allergy by an astute pediatric specialist, survived on a diet that consisted primarily of lamb, rice, and occasional bananas. Ensuring that no products containing milk ingredients entered their home required constant vigilance, and Weissman worried about "becoming one of those mothers who are all about their children—or child" and unintentionally turning her son into a demanding and capricious, spoiled and stubborn, individual.[10]

Striking a balance between the heightened attentiveness required to prevent allergens from entering an allergic child's environment, and the desire to bring such children and their siblings up as normally as possible, may create unexpected problems—a point illustrated by the time that Weissman left Eden at home with her mother-in-law, so that she could take her daughter to a birthday party. When Weissman returned one hour later, she found Eden scratching his neck. "He needs to eat, but I waited" to feed him, explained her mother-in-law.[11] When the liquid Benadryl, administered on the advice of their physician, failed to reverse the allergic reaction underway, Eden's hands puffed up like two tiny baseball gloves. They phoned the doctor again, and he advised getting Eden to an emergency room as quickly as possible.

Weissman and her mother-in-law threw a coat over Eden's shoulders to shield him from the bitter January cold in New York City and hailed a cab. She remembers that the taxi ride to the emergency room seemed to take forever, and in route Eden began scratching himself all over. When he lifted his shirt, they saw hives of various sizes on his stomach and sides covered in red marks from Eden's persistent scratching.[12] When his lips and eyelids began to swell, Weissman panicked. Fortunately, the emergency room was not busy, and Eden was quickly treated with epinephrine. His diagnosis upon discharge: anaphylaxis—cause unknown.[13] Idiopathic anaphylaxis, a form of the disease in which triggers cannot be identified despite a detailed history and careful diagnostic assessment, remains relatively rare.[14] When a child has an anaphylactic reaction after all known allergens have been removed from the home environment, that allergic response raises already heightened levels of concern about the health and well-being of that young person. Feeding Eden was a difficult enough task when the anaphylactic triggers were identifiable.

After this incident, Weissman realized that even well-controlled allergies could erupt at any moment, and it changed the way her entire family lived. They toted epinephrine auto-injectors, inhalers, and antihistamines everywhere, and they limited their travels. She learned to accept the fact that her fear of accidental exposures and cross-contamination would linger into the foreseeable future, and she worried that someday she might read a food label too quickly and expose Eden to danger.[15] She wondered if she and her partner would buckle under the effort that it took to maintain constant watchfulness over a child with multiple food allergies (to dairy, eggs, soy, nuts, fish, shellfish, and several fruits) who had also developed asthma at the age of three. She hoped that Eden might outgrow some of his allergies, that there might eventually be an effective treatment or cure, and that he would avoid a premature death and live long enough to make a full contribution to society.[16]

-◊-

Lisa Collins, a family therapist whose son suffers from peanut allergies, recognizes that having a child with a serious health concern is among the worst things that can happen to parents.[17] When doctors explained to her that he just needed to avoid peanuts to remain healthy, she found that advice well-meaning, but ultimately unhelpful, particularly when friends and family members shared stories with her of allergic individuals dying after consuming a food allergen. Collins found that parents had to grapple with the realization that everyone involved with the care and upbringing of their son must be educated about the severity of his condition—even though he remained symptom-free until triggered.[18] Some people around him struggled to grasp the severity of the allergic response, while others only half believed it, suspecting exaggeration from worried parents. Still others dismissed their concerns altogether—most hurtfully, members of their own extended family. As a result of that range of responses, people like Collins spend an inordinate amount of time worrying about their child's safety at daycare, at the neighbor's house, and even at granddad's place.[19]

Collins recalls having to factor her son's peanut allergy into almost every decision-making process throughout her day, and she frequently imagined worst-case scenarios (the cookies and milk offered by hosts, the peanut crackers other children brought as a snack to school, kids trading foods, cross-contact in cafeterias, an allergic reaction missed by a busy teacher leading to delayed treatment). Like other people with severely food-allergic children, thoughts such as these flooded her mind: Will my child have safe meals at school? Will someone know how to recognize and to treat an allergic reaction? Will an epinephrine auto-injector be always available for my child? Is the emergency room close by?[20] Parents struggling to balance these and other concerns may be perceived as overprotective, though they seek to ensure their child's well-being.

In addition, it can be difficult for parents of food-allergic children to encourage their independence and normality when high levels of alertness are required to ensure safe eating environments. Billy, for example, once paged his mother to pick him up at school after he saw kids eating peanuts in his classroom. When she arrived, Billy's mother took him to lunch at a nearby restaurant, where they had eaten before, and she kept him out of school for the rest of the day.[21] Allergy and asthma-related behaviors in children may either be positively reinforced, by getting their way, by receiving privileges, and by gaining attention—or through negative reinforcement by allowing them to escape school, chores, and other responsibilities. In some families, non-food-allergic siblings may develop feelings of jealousy, anger, and bitterness toward their parents or the sick child for requiring extra attention: when certain foods are prohibited in the home; when vacation destinations are limited and trips shortened; and when important celebrations such as birthday parties are curtailed.[22]

Correlations also exist between overprotective parenting and the development of social problems in food-allergic children among their peers.[23] For this reason, Collins believes that children should begin taking age-appropriate control of their own allergies by asking adults before eating anything. In her view, school-age children must learn on their own to negotiate cafeterias, field trips, slumber parties, and bus rides that may expose them to allergens. This is a frightening proposition for many parents, and Collins warns that the "letting-go" process can be particularly difficult when children from ages 5 to 11 years old are just learning to read food labels, to communicate with others about their food allergies, and to take responsibility for carrying epinephrine and learning how to self-administer it.[24] Some parents of allergic children report being worried, frustrated, exhausted, unable to sleep, and physically and emotionally drained. These difficulties often lead them to restrict the social lives of their other children, a move that upon reflection may give rise to feelings of self-doubt concerning their parenting abilities.[25]

New sets of challenges await caregivers, family members, and friends of children with food allergies as they grow up. Preteens and teens are more likely to conceal or to minimize their allergies and to exhibit riskier eating without planning for possible emergencies, particularly at social events involving food and during overnight excursions.[26] As they grow towards independence, preteens and teens will still depend on others for assistance, especially during allergic reactions when they are physically unable to help themselves. They tend to lean on parents and primary caregivers most, but in managing daily life with severe food allergies, preteens and teens also seek assistance from friends, support through social media, and the care of those who understand their unusual needs. Studies show that many teens with food-induced anaphylaxis calculate risks by engaging in activities that they regarded as dangerous when they had epinephrine auto-injectors on hand.[27] Some protected themselves by leaving places or events that they considered too risky, and they turned to trusted friends to keep them safe and to shield them from socially devastating situations, such as anaphylaxis in a public place. Although they sometimes took unnecessary risks to avoid embarrassing situations, they also refused to participate in social activities with peers who did not face the same limitations.[28]

As a teenager, I began adopting risk-based food strategies after eating that cookie at Angela's house and enduring rebound anaphylaxis. Because my childhood food allergies began with relatively mild symptoms (vomiting, hives, and that "fist in the stomach" feeling), my parents relied on me to navigate social activities involving food, to scrutinize labels, and to monitor my own nutritional intake. When those allergic reactions became anaphylactic in my teens, I assumed responsibility for what I ate and learned to keep to myself most of the apprehension about food that assailed me. Although many parents and caregivers instill the need for constant vigilance in young people with food allergies, the time will come when they must accept the fact that it's simply impossible for children, preteens, and teens to control every aspect of their lives involving food—and to accept the fact that there will always be life-threatening risks beyond anyone's control.

Preteens and teens often have good reason not to disclose their food allergies—many of which carry over into adulthood: the fear of being misunderstood, the fear of becoming the subject of unwanted attention, the fear of trusting others with such a disclosure. Studies of other chronic health conditions suggest that boys have more difficulty coping with food allergies, since from childhood into adulthood males are more likely than females to perceive chronic illnesses (e.g., asthma, diabetes, food allergies) as a sign of weakness, to conceal their diagnoses and symptoms, and to exhibit problems adapting to illness management.[29] Parents may unwittingly contribute to their social anxiety by modeling worry and attempting to control their food choices. Adolescents often feel acute embarrassment over the attention given to them by peers, teachers, parents, and others concerned with their well-being. Such interventions can be mortifying for teenagers and young adults, especially when they have already begun to manage their own food allergies.[30]

Nonetheless, families and teachers play enormous supporting roles in the lives of food-allergic preteens and teens. Thirteen-year-old Adrian, who suffers from a severe nut allergy, observed that at his mom's house, "we never ever have anything with nuts in it," though his "little brother can have sweets sometimes, but never anything with nuts." At his father's place, Adrian knows that there are probably "a bit more" nuts around, but that overall "when Mum and Dad cook I feel almost completely safe."[31] As a teenager living with anaphylaxis, Adrian cautiously regards his parents' homes as something of a "safe-zone" for eating, though he also must remain alert in both places. Likewise, Isabella gradually learned how to self-manage her allergy to milk protein: "When I was little it was mum and dad who knew everything, without them I was helpless, but now I feel that I can look after myself, I know that I can't eat certain things." She looks forward to a time when she has her own apartment, and she plans to stock it with "everything milk-free."[32]

Of course, every family situation is different, and living with someone with food-induced anaphylaxis involves constant accommodation. When parents view making such adjustments as a burden, teenagers and young adults must remind family members, and the people that they interact with most frequently, about their allergies and explain to them what to do in an emergency. It's incumbent upon older children to make sure that they check food products and travel with necessary medications. Whereas parents of young allergic children tend to lend their support in managing food-induced anaphylaxis, and to act as liaisons with schools and other educational institutions to make sure that necessary support is given without stigmatizing their child, adolescents and young adults must learn to handle social activities involving food to protect themselves.[33] Parents, grandparents, and caregivers who witness an allergic reaction in a child may become overprotective and experience greater anxiety than parents of non-allergic children, but there is also great joy in watching such a child grow into an independent person.[34]

-◊-

After anaphylaxis, children of all ages can develop fears about future exposures to allergens, which can result in avoidance of social events involving food, including extracurricular activities, sleepovers at friends', and participation in school field trips.[35] Such behaviors hinder the development of adaptive coping skills, diminish social self-confidence, and inhibit the growth of healthy interpersonal relationships. Fourteen-year-old Joel has learned to inform new folks at school about his allergy, and he remembers to pack epinephrine autoinjectors, but that does not keep him from imagining lying unconscious as school officials search for his locker key among his pockets, thus wasting precious time getting to his medications. "I don't think it'll be like that," Joel admits, but "it's just that it can happen."[36] Sixteen-year-old Joanna figured out how to deal with the unpredictability of accidental exposures by accepting that any day "could be that day."[37] Even with that understanding, she reported a persistent fear of death associated with being unable to breathe. The question of when to seek counseling for unrelenting fears comes down to the degree to which phobias and anxieties manifest themselves in physically and socially unhealthful avoidance behaviors.

As soon as practicable, preteens and teenagers should discuss food allergies with doctors, peers, school officials, and restaurant staff on their own terms. David, a 14-year-old student with allergies to milk protein and eggs, goes straight to the school kitchen to retrieve allergen-free meals prepared especially for him, though sometimes he must sit alone to eat them.[38] Alva, a 15-year-old who self-manages her allergies to peas and milk, used to sit alone at a cafeteria table reserved for her, which she always wiped down first as a precaution. Eventually, she learned to enjoy sitting with understanding friends at lunch and to pack instant noodles in the event of an unplanned after-school visit to someone's house. She knows that she can't eat dinner with her friends' families, but she and her friends can at least eat noodles together. "I don't like eating different food, I want to eat the same as the others," she admits, tacitly acknowledging that food connects people together in important ways.[39]

In place of allergy-safe meals prepared by doting relatives and guardians in childhood, one must realize that cross-contamination from knives, spoons, spatulas, bowls, and cutting boards is always possible, as is the spread of allergens in kitchen prep areas. Because eating away from home always involves some danger, fears of cross-contact are the most difficult to root out of the mind, especially given that they serve an important self-preservation function. I remember when my friend Michael's mother and aunt made homemade peach ice cream for me. I was overly cautious in refusing to try it, though I would have loved to, and probably could have done so without incident. Knowing they baked with tree nuts (stashed in the kitchen) made it easy for me to imagine a moment of inattentiveness during preparation, or even nut protein residue in the ice cream machine from a prior batch of butter pecan. From their house to the nearest emergency room took 20 to 30 minutes, so I weighed that risk as well.

-◊-

Just as concerned friends, family members, and peers may positively impact the lives of people living with food allergies, bullies, "frenemies," malevolent rivals, and others with self-serving intentions may inflict on them harmful and enduring consequences. In a 2010 survey of more than 350 teens and young adults, researchers at Mount Sinai Medical Center found that approximately one in four school-age children are bullied, teased, or harassed because of their food allergy. Nearly 60 percent of those surveyed reported being touched or threatened by a food allergen—*and more than 20 percent cited teachers or school staff as perpetrators!*[40] Zac, for instance, recalls being harassed "mostly by adults, but in some instances, by peers. In the fifth grade, my new teacher (who was fully aware of my 504 plan) selected me as part of a science experiment involving peanut butter and even though I reminded her of my allergy, peanut butter was rubbed on my hands during the experiment."[41] In the seventh grade, Zac continued, "one student found out about my allergy and where my locker was, as well as my combination. He put peanut butter inside the locker, outside the locker, and on the back of the lock."[42]

Children and young adults with food allergies can also experience taunting and bullying for having to carry emergency medication and for receiving special treatment at school. Victims of bullying face feelings of insecurity, anxiety, depression, as well as a lack of self-esteem and increased suicidal ideation that inhibits their ability to concentrate in school and results in avoidance behaviors.[43] Although deaths related to food-bullying are rare, when allergic people are touched with an allergen, or when that allergen is secretly introduced into their food, it poses a significant danger. In 2017, a 13-year-old student died after having an anaphylactic reaction to a piece of cheese forced on him by a fellow student at a West London school. The victim, Karanbir Cheema, had a care plan in place, and the executive head teacher reported that although it was followed, Karanbir died after ten days in intensive care. As his father explained to one newspaper reporter, my son had food allergies, "but he was very careful." Yet, we "had to watch him die." No parent, he insisted, "should have to go through that."[44] His mother, who did not know that Karanbir was being bullied, sent him to school on the morning of the incident never expecting "it to be the last goodbye."[45] For allegedly flicking cheese toward the unfortunate boy's mouth, police arrested one of Karanbir's classmates on suspicion of attempted murder.

Reports of bullying based on race, color, and disability in school appear in the media daily, and the rise of allergy bullying worries some experts.[46] Many food-allergic adolescents express concern about having to explain their condition to others because it may result in social mortification and encourage bullying. The verbal, physical, social, and psychological bullying of allergic people usually involves a power imbalance manipulated by a bully, or group of bullies, toward one or more persons with an intention to harm. The taunting and harassing of children and adolescents with food allergies is not limited to a particular country or region, and it universally coincides with feelings of embarrassment, of being different from everybody else, and of being left out of activities because of a medical condition. One comprehensive examination of school-age children in Italy, which distinguished allergy-related bullying from general bullying, found food-allergic students twice as likely to be bullied.[47] These and other findings suggest the need for medical practitioners to discuss the elevated risk of bullying and intimidation in school with patients and to encourage parents to advocate for their food-allergic children.

Bullying also takes place during school-related activities that involve travel and overnight stays. Brandon, a 16-year-old American with an allergy to eggs, became a target of food-bullying on a trip with his bowling team. Diagnosed with a life-threatening allergy at the age of one, Williams recalled the time when one of his teammates decided to eat a fast-food sandwich on Brandon's hotel bed and spilled mayonnaise on the comforter and on Brandon's jacket. When Brandon asked him not to eat on his bed, the teammate merely smiled and shoved the mayonnaise-laden sandwich in Williams' face. Brandon reported that it was common for people at school to wave food that he couldn't eat near him, and he acknowledged the undercurrent of risk inherent in such bullying. "It wouldn't be funny to break someone's arm to send them to the hospital," Williams observed. "Why would it be funny to send someone to the hospital for an allergy?"[48]

In 2014, lead author Rachel Annunziato wrote that her research team had discovered considerably more food-bullying than expected. It did not matter how serious the allergy was, or whether the targets of bullying were allergic to peanuts, wheat, or shellfish. One third of students interviewed experienced food-bullying at school *more than twice a month*. One child's mother conjectured that it's simply human nature "to find cracks and attack there."[49] That recognition of weakness and vulnerability keeps some patients from disclosing their condition where it might otherwise be helpful to do so. It's wonderful that increased awareness of food allergies among parents, school officials, and the general public has resulted in the formulation of 504 Plans to accommodate students' needs and the establishment of "nut-free" zones, but these developments do little to discourage the bullying that begins as early as first or second grade when kids begin to hone in on differences between themselves and their classmates, yet lack the ability to think through the implications of their actions.

Several advocacy organizations—including the Allergy & Asthma Network, Food Allergy & Anaphylaxis Connection Team, and Kids with Food Allergies—sponsored an anti-bullying campaign in 2017 publicizing the message that food-bullying can prove fatal. The following year, Sony Pictures was forced to apologize for a scene in *Peter Rabbit*, a film based loosely on a 1902 book written by Beatrix Potter, in which the villain Tom McGregor is discovered to suffer from an allergy to blackberries. In the offending scene, the rabbits throw blackberries into Tom's mouth. As he enters anaphylactic shock, Tom turns red, injects himself with epinephrine, and the rabbits celebrate their "victory."[50] In this way, the film depicts food-bullying in a manner that makes light of severe allergic reactions.

Although controversial for many reasons, attacks on food-allergic kids in high school and college increasingly carry legal repercussions for perpetrators. In January 2018, a 14-year-old girl from Pennsylvania faced felony charges of aggravated assault; she had rubbed a known allergen (pineapple) on one of her hands and high-fived a girl with an allergy to that food.[51] Five months earlier, a Central Michigan University student pleaded guilty to assault and battery after being charged with smearing peanut butter on the face of an unconscious student with a known peanut allergy.[52] Even more terrifying for people with food-induced anaphylaxis, civil lawsuits have been filed against restaurants accused of *deliberately putting allergens into food ordered by customers who made their allergies known when ordering*. In one such case in Massachusetts, a father filed a lawsuit on behalf of his daughter who experienced an allergic reaction after eating a grilled cheese sandwich with peanut butter hidden inside it, even though the family explicitly noted the peanut allergy in an online order form. One of the lawyers representing the family highlighted the long-term psychological repercussions of that kind of bullying, noting that after taking a bite, she asked her parents in a panic, "Am I going to die?"[53] Such occurrences instill fear in victims that persist into adulthood and manifest in social isolation at gatherings where unsafe foods are present.

When students with food allergies have milk poured over them, mayonnaise waved in their faces, cake thrown at them, peanut butter smeared on their bodies, their food surreptitiously contaminated with an allergen, life-threatening reactions cannot always be resolved by the prompt use of epinephrine auto-injectors, as the Karanbir Cheema case demonstrates. Bullies target peers with food allergies because managing diet is a daily visible struggle, and the steps these young people must take to stay alive (such as eating at separate tables) alienates them and provides openings for bullies to tease and harass. The Cleveland Clinic advises allergic victims to assertively tell bullies to stop, to contact an adult in charge, and to inform parents about harassment immediately.[54] A buddy system should be put in place for support, and an action plan activated when allergic reactions occur.

When food-bullying results in emotional distress, victims and their parents might consider psychological and nutritional counseling, which can have positive lifelong consequences. A counselor can help children and parents to understand the importance of the strict elimination of allergens from the diet while ensuring that patients meet the caloric and protein needs of growing bodies. A nutritionist might offer insight into what foods can be safely substituted for allergens eliminated, determine if vitamin and mineral supplementation are necessary, and help with meal planning.[55] Supportive counseling from primary care physicians includes educating patients on the differences between food intolerance and food allergy, debunking myths (such as it's okay to have a taste of something to see if it's safe), discussing the nature of anaphylaxis, probing for co-existing conditions like asthma, addressing unproven treatments, and finding optimal strategies for preventing exposure to allergens.

As essential as these strategies have proven, psychological counseling might also become part of learning to live with life-threatening food allergies. As children enter adolescence and young adulthood with less external oversight regarding their food choices, they are less likely to read labels or to ask about ingredients in restaurants before eating. As they move into adulthood, they sometimes hide the extent of their illness so as not to stand out or to appear sickly. In the workplace, they can thrive when colleagues and peers focus on their personal and professional qualities, rather than on their medical condition. Young people may easily feel acute embarrassment about what happens to their bodies during an anaphylactic reaction and develop a lack of trust in the outside world regarding food. A good counselor might ask such individuals to re-imagine the event that triggered anaphylaxis and to put their thoughts and feelings into words.[56]

Survivors of anaphylaxis can be emotionally affected by that terrifying experience in a number of ways, from acute embarrassment for disrupting a party to profound skepticism about the safety of food one is served. When thoughts and fearful emotions about what happened to the body during anaphylaxis become obsessive and incongruent with the severity of those allergic emergencies, counseling may help to resolve maladaptive emotions that linger long after allergic reactions are over. Emotion-focused therapy helps people who might otherwise push a problematic experience from conscious awareness to move past trauma in an adaptive way by revealing maladaptive emotions and their hidden meanings.[57] People who feel disappointed or disgusted with themselves for not checking labels or asking about ingredients, or who minimize the severity of a reaction so as not to foster guilt in a friend or a family member, may find relief in examining such emotions from different angles.

Anaphylactic reactions can also trigger acute stress disorder three to 30 days after the event. When that stress response occurs more than a month afterward, which is common in my experience, it may result in PTSD.[58] It has been more than 20 years since my last dance with anaphylaxis, and I'm still hypervigilant and sometimes unnecessarily fearful around food and some beverages. The American Psychological Association recognized anaphylaxis as a trigger for PTSD in 2013, but it will take more research to formulate empirically driven approaches to working with trauma in food-allergic children and adults.[59] A medical family therapy approach (in which integrated health care teams address the physical, emotional, spiritual, and relational needs of patients) makes counselors part of a group of doctors, nurses, nutritionists, and other professionals who can bridge the gap between addressing patients' physiological and psychological needs. In this way, medical professionals can help the food-allergic to better cope with the daily challenges of living with life-threatening allergies.

-◊-

As an adult with food-induced anaphylaxis, I depend on other people all the time—often at considerable cost to those closest to me. Savannah quit eating tree nuts, a favorite childhood food, after we met. She sometimes keeps nutty foods in her office, as a snack in between meals, but she's careful not to bring food home that could be dangerous. Because she does most of the cooking, and I do most of the housework, she must read labels in the grocery store, re-read them at home, and put up with my repeated queries: "Did you read the label?" Recently, she inadvertently brought home food containing one of these vague, but all too common, warnings:

> "May contain peanuts."
> "This product was produced in a facility that also processes peanuts."
> "Made on equipment that also processes peanuts and tree nuts."
> "May contain traces of tree nuts."

Even though the Food and Drug Administration warns that these advisory labels should not be used by manufacturers "as a substitute for adhering to current good manufacturing practices and must be truthful and not misleading," I avoid foods with such labeling.[60] It seems clear that many companies include such language to reduce their liability in our litigious society.

Be that as it may, a few years ago we both accidentally bought products in the grocery store that included this kind of labeling. Savannah picked up a shortcake that contained no nuts, but had a nebulous warning about allergens, and I grabbed a package of Thomas's English

Muffins without reading the label first, because I ate them as a child. Savannah spotted the allergy warning label before opening the package. After reading it, I went to the company website (in late 2018) and found the following statement:

> We assure you that we adhere to Good Manufacturing Practices as established by the FDA. We take abundant precaution to prevent cross contact of allergenic ingredients between batches, and our bakeries are inspected to ensure that they meet or exceed all regulatory and baking industry standards. We understand that highly sensitive consumers need to know when there is even the remotest possibility of inadvertent cross contact of allergenic ingredients during processing. To that end we disclose that the following allergenic ingredients are used in some of our manufacturing facilities and that inadvertent cross contact is remotely possible: milk, eggs, soy, almonds, walnuts, peanuts and hazelnuts (filberts). Wheat is used in all of our facilities and all of our products as an ingredient. Please refer to ingredient labels on our products for full disclosure of the ingredients used in that product.

This example shows that food allergens sometimes lurk in unexpected places. On this occasion, we could joke about our mistake. If those muffins had contained tree nuts, and I hadn't seen the warning, or chose to ignore it, the outcome might have been quite different.

Nearly all baked goods made in-house at our local grocery store—as well as the cheese and deli meats sliced there—contain warnings such as this one: "Allergens: May contain crustacean shellfish, eggs, fish, milk, peanuts, soy, tree nuts, and wheat due to shared preparation area." These days, I seek out prepackaged food items without such warnings. Another difficulty that I encounter when reading food labels (and sometimes menus in restaurants) is identifying unfamiliar ingredients. Recently, I bought a frozen entrée that sat in the freezer for months until Savannah ate it because it contained cooked red quinoa, which I didn't feel comfortable eating even after researching it online (it's a flowering plant botanically related to spinach). Savannah once purchased pasta containing truffles, and the little black dots on the noodles gave me concern, even though truffles are essentially mushrooms. It took a while before I was willing to try it, and then did so only reluctantly. Such instances highlight lingering, sometimes irrational, fears of unknown foods among survivors of anaphylaxis.

Having grown up a sickly kid who was picky about food, I confess to being difficult to feed even without the tree nut allergy. I trust only a handful of people to cook because they take my condition seriously. Mom eats tree nuts, but she puts them away when I visit, cleans countertops with bleach, and puts a label on anything that I should avoid—even items made with a bag of flour that she might have had open while cooking with tree nuts. I rely on John, the son of a retired English professor from my department, to cook without nuts when he invites us over. I depend on Art, a former military policeman and building contractor to read food labels carefully, something he had never done before. After seeing the overdose scene in the film *Pulp Fiction* (1994), he jokes that someday he hopes to get the opportunity to stab me in the heart with an epinephrine auto-injector—and I never fail to remind him that epinephrine auto-injectors are delivered intramuscularly into the thigh! Another thing I appreciate about Art, he often leaves food labels out for me to read before we eat.

When turning down other invitations to dinner, I generally cite my allergy, and will instead ask those folks over to our place for a meal. That decision, however, places a burden on Savannah, and because of her busy work schedule, we often miss opportunities to meet new friends. I can't participate in the community dinners at the eco-village co-housing neighborhood where we live either. Even with a couple of children in residence with food-induced anaphylaxis, and lots of food intolerances (particularly to gluten) among adults, I pass on them due to cross-contact on knives, baking sheets, and cutting boards on which tree nuts are frequently chopped, and because prep areas can get messy. I could request nut-free meals but hesitate to inconvenience others to accommodate one person. In any case, one can never be sure how mindful the cooks will be. The other day, I volunteered to wash dishes after a group meal. One of the cooks knew of my allergy and assured me that there were no nuts in that evening meal, but I encountered left-over walnuts when washing a large salad bowl by hand. Not surprisingly, when this person offered to prepare a community meal with me in mind, I politely declined! People often mean well, but they frequently fail to distinguish mild food intolerances from life-threatening food allergies. Savannah appreciates healthy food and fellowship, and so she joins community meals without me.

When Arno and Sabine invited us to visit them in the south of France, where they were living after another stint in China, they realized that much had changed in terms of the sometimes reckless eating habits I had adopted in Shanghai. To allay some angst about traveling in a country where I couldn't speak the language, they took a train to Paris to meet us at the airport. We stayed for a night or two in the capital and visited the customary sites: the Eiffel Tower, Arc de Triomphe,

Louvre Museum, Champs-Élysées. On our first night, they found a sea-food restaurant with little threat from tree nuts, but from that moment onward, every meal we took together would be impacted by my presence. All bakeries were out, due to the ubiquity of tree nuts, and even plain baguettes could have cross-contact with allergens. Cheese and sausage ingredients had to be scrutinized, since they sometimes contain nuts. During the day, I gravitated toward fast food joints that served hamburgers and fries, which left everyone else free to eat where they wanted.

We left Paris in a small Hyundai crossover vehicle rented for the trip, and on the way south stopped for one night at Sabine's parents' home, a converted farmhouse in the Burgundy countryside that had been passed down through her family for generations. Since it was far from a hospital emergency room, strict avoidance was crucial, but her parents understood and prepared delicious homemade bread and fresh goat cheese that, along with red wine, kept me going. After arriving at Arno's parents' place, which overlooked the Mediterranean, our hosts planned three safe meals per day for me and vigilantly kept tree nuts (and products made with them) out of the kitchen. Although we all pitched in to help cook and clean up, my presence meant scrutinizing food labels, altering recipes, and making bread instead of buying it. Even with those precautions, I stuck with a few foods that I felt comfortable eating, though others were safe too.

When our visit ended, and we headed back to Paris alone, Arno wrote a letter in French that explained my food allergy to restaurant personnel. Savannah prepared a couple of meals, one of which I ate before going to a fancy restaurant in an historic chateau, where I had a couple of glasses of wine as she dined. It's hard to fully express my gratitude to Arno's family, to Bill and Afifi, to Giuseppe and his parents, and to my friends and family members for their constant accommodation—without which I could not easily get along. I hate being the center of unwanted attention wherever food is being prepared and eaten, the awkward outsider when people gather around food, the "problem person who disrupts things for others," as singer Mandy Harvey puts it.[61] But, until the time comes when doctors and scientists develop effective treatments, those of us with food allergies must depend on the goodwill of friends and family members who sacrifice in so many ways to protect us.

-◊-

Chapter Four. Upon Others, Our Lives Depend

There currently exists no cure for severe food allergies, but Scott Sicherer believes that the "future looks bright" for new therapies.[62] The Food and Drug Administration recently approved Palforzia, an oral immunotherapy regimen, to treat peanut allergy in children. That drug reduces the risk that an accidental exposure to small amounts of peanut will set off a life-threatening response. Palforzia reduces sensitivity to peanuts by gradually exposing children to small amounts of peanut protein over the course of six months, until they can safely eat the equivalent of two peanuts. Because that treatment regime is not always effective and includes serious possible side effects, the Food and Drug Administration will require that initial and increased doses be delivered at a medical facility capable of treating anaphylaxis, will restrict the drug to patients who agree to always carry epinephrine, and will include a warning that patients must still avoid peanuts.[63]

Palforzia treats young people 4 to 17 years of age and just for peanut allergy, and it remains effective only if patients continue to consume small, prescribed amounts of the allergen. Although people with multiple food allergies stand to benefit little from this innovative treatment, because deaths from anaphylaxis occur from peanuts more than any other food, the introduction of trace amounts of peanut protein followed by maintenance dosages may allow some allergic people to travel with less fear, eat in restaurants with reduced anxiety, and participate in more social events around food. The fact that after one year, two-thirds of the nearly 400 children who received the Palforzia treatment tolerated the equivalent of two peanuts without having an allergic reaction is encouraging news,[64] but there's a long way to go before food-allergic people will be able to live normal lives, as the following review of current treatment modalities demonstrates.

Approaches to treating allergies may be divided into allergen-specific and non–allergen-specific therapies. Allergen-specific therapies (better known as allergy shots) provide allergists and immunologists with an effective treatment for common conditions such as allergic rhinitis, allergic asthma, and stinging insect hypersensitivity.[65] This form of therapy typically involves the administration of gradually increasing quantities of a patient's relevant allergens (usually through the skin) until a dose is reached that is effective in inducing tolerance, decreasing symptoms, and preventing disease recurrence. Ideally effective allergen-specific therapies for food allergies would gradually increase doses of a culprit food allergen, without triggering an adverse immune response to the therapy itself, and eventually allow the food to be consumed in normal quantities with no symptoms. By contrast, non–allergen-specific (or immune-modulating) therapies aim to create a state of tolerance by altering the global host immune response of the body, rather than addressing reactions tied to a specific allergen.[66] In this way, patients could be treated for multiple food allergies with a single therapy by using, for example, anti–IgE antibodies to interrupt inflammatory signals.

Allergen-specific therapies have long seemed like a promising approach for their ability to create desensitization to, or tolerance of, allergens. "Desensitization" refers to a temporary, reversible state wherein patients may ingest a higher dose of an antigen without any symptoms when compared with the pretreatment-tolerated dose.[67] The lengthy periods of time needed to obtain desensitization—and the danger of generating "significant adverse events" (i.e., anaphylaxis) during trials—currently limits their use for food allergy.[68] One might imagine joining a clinical trial aimed at boosting tolerance to an antigen by introducing increasing amounts of a food extract, only to have it trigger anaphylaxis, the very outcome that people like me fear most: not being able to breathe after eating. The tragic death of nine-year-old Brooklyn Secor, who had asthma and was allergic to dairy products, from anaphylaxis in May 2021—while she was participating in dairy desensitization therapy—highlights the limitations and dangers of trying to gradually increase food allergen tolerance.[69]

Because of the possibility of adverse reactions during allergen-specific immunotherapy, researchers are investigating multiple routes of antigen delivery, including under the skin, topically on the skin, under the tongue, as well as through the mouth. Subcutaneous (under the skin) immunotherapy involves long and tedious protocols, such as weekly injections during a build-up phase, followed by monthly maintenance injections for a period of three-to-five years.[70] The efficacy of this approach has been demonstrated for allergic conditions such as hay fever, but in the case of food allergies, the risk of potentially deadly reactions may make it an unsuitable treatment modality. Epicutaneous immunotherapy, involving the application of an allergen-containing patch on the skin, has been shown to increase threshold levels in peanut-allergic patients, especially children. In one study, adverse reactions occurring in application sites remained mostly local (erythema and eczema), and were visible for several days, which suggests that epicutaneous immunotherapy may be safer than other immunotherapies.[71]

Sublingual immunotherapy involves the administering of small drops of an allergen extract (in doses ranging from micrograms to milligrams) held under the tongue for two minutes and then swallowed. This method of treating food allergies often takes place in phases: a build-up phase consisting of weekly to biweekly dose escalations administered until a target dose is reached, followed by a second maintenance phase in which the patient self-administers daily home doses over the course of months or years. Hopeful results from this approach include peanut, milk, hazelnut, and peach allergies. In one instance, peanut allergic children underwent four months of dose escalation, followed by eight months of maintenance dosing, and safely ingested twenty times more peanut protein than the placebo group.[72] While not a cure, raising the allergic threshold would provide a safeguard against accidental ingestion and relieve a good deal of trepidation around trace peanut cross-contamination. Although it provides a better safety profile, the fact that only half of 24 subjects treated with sublingual immunotherapy for peanut allergy for five years achieved sustained unresponsiveness suggests that it is less effective than oral immunotherapy in inducing desensitization.[73]

Oral immunotherapies (like Palforzia) generally involve the gradual administration of small amounts of an allergen mixed with a food vehicle over the course of several months to years. Such procedures may include an initial rapid dose escalation (i.e., six-to-eight doses of the allergen over one or two days) followed by a build-up phase of about six-to-12 months until a target dose is reached. Afterwards, a maintenance phase, lasting several months or years, can be conducted at home. To test permanence of protection, participants halt maintenance doses for one-to-three months, followed by a "tolerance" food challenge. Oral food allergen dosing creates a lot of apprehension in participants, especially about mild symptoms that are not very concerning from a medical perspective. When clinicians told patients that these mild reactions offered a positive sign that the immune system was working, participants seemed to get through the desensitization process more easily—and with less fear.[74]

In addition to these advances, positive Phase I data from a clinical trial evaluating the safety of a new peanut allergy vaccine is generating hope among those with food allergies. By using antigen fragments, rather than whole peanut allergens, the vaccine (PVX108) targets allergen-specific T-cells and promotes tolerance with fewer harmful reactions. In a double-blind, placebo-controlled study, researchers observed the effects of single, ascending doses of the vaccine over a 16-week period with only mild to moderately severe adverse effects.[75]

Another allergen-specific immunotherapy (HAL-MPE) that consists of natural peanut allergen extract, chemically modified to limit allergenicity, also shows promise in Phase I.[76]

In terms of non–allergen-specific therapies, anti–IgE treatments currently work well for moderate to severe asthma and persistent hives with an unknown cause (chronic idiopathic urticaria) by preventing the rapid onset of symptoms (coughing, wheezing, nasal congestion, hives and swelling) triggered by the body's production of IgE, which attaches to antigens and initiates an allergic reaction. Studies show that while some people experience no improvement, others undergoing anti–IgE therapy could tolerate more of a food allergen. Unfortunately, this treatment can sometimes also trigger allergic reactions.[77] Probiotics (live microorganisms that confer a health benefit) and prebiotics (nutrients that help healthy bacteria grow) may ultimately prove beneficial in the treatment of food allergies, especially if the hygiene hypothesis proves correct.[78] That theory posits that clean living environments deprive the immune system of a proper target and make it more likely to attack harmless food proteins. A similar line of thinking applies to parasites, which might be used to redirect immune responses to food proteins, given that people living in parasitized regions of the world tend to have fewer allergies. While both approaches require further research, early studies suggest that effective treatments for food allergies may lie elsewhere.

Having lived in China, I'm intrigued by the herbal approach founded on the principles of Traditional Chinese Medicine developed by Dr. Xiu Min Li at Mount Sinai. She has devised an herbal formula based on the symptoms that one develops from food allergies, which has proven effective in mice with peanut allergy by allowing them to consume the allergen beyond the treatment period. When the allergy began to recur, retreatment with herbs protected the mice again. The challenge seems to lie in narrowing the number of ingredients in the formula to find those most efficacious and to reduce the large number of herbal pills per day currently prescribed for treatment. In her Manhattan clinic, Li treats allergic people with herbal-compounded medicines used for eczema, asthma, and food allergy. In addition to other Traditional Chinese Medicine practices such as acupuncture, Dr. Li gives her patients tablets to take orally, teas to drink, and body creams to use topically. Families come to her from all over the world in hopes that she can either cure their children of food allergies, or at least reduce their allergic sensitivity, so that they may enjoy a better quality of life.[79]

After tolerating all types of nuts her entire life, Anarie Matchett developed food-induced anaphylaxis to peanuts and tree nuts at the age of 14. Her worst reaction occurred during a canoe trip near Lake Huron after she ate pita bread and entered full-blown anaphylaxis on the water. Her camp counselor administered four epinephrine auto-injectors in succession to keep her alive until firefighters could reach her by canoe. Once in the ambulance, they rushed her to the hospital. Anarie survived due to the efforts of her counselor, the rapid response by rescuers, and the work of the emergency room team. Her mother, desperate to help her daughter find a treatment, sought out Dr. Li.

To rebalance the immune system over time, Dr. Li designs treatments using herbs to prevent memory cells from producing allergy antibodies and to reverse IgE sensitization in her patients over time. Despite successes with people such as Anarie, who accidentally ate a pastry containing nuts while studying abroad in France—and didn't have a reaction, a paper published in the *Journal of Allergy and Clinical Immunology* found the herbs no more effective than the placebo.[80] Anarie, who continued her studies in Amsterdam, can eat nuts now. Perhaps one reason for the clinical failure, suggests Dr. Li, is that in her private practice she designs treatment protocols for each patient and closely monitors dosages, something not possible in formal trials.

Writing for the journal *Allergy, Asthma & Clinical Immunology*, Dr. Li and her fellow researchers asserted that combined Traditional Chinese Medicine therapy successfully prevented anaphylaxis in three pediatric patients with extraordinarily frequent and potentially life-threatening food allergies.[81] She believes that some protocols may be standardized in the future, so that patients will not have to travel to New York City to see her. Similarly, researchers at Gifu University in Japan advocate for the medical treatment of food allergies with personalized medicine tailored to each patient, like those being pioneered for the treatment of cancer. They argue that because biomarkers, clinical symptoms, and genetics vary from patient to patient—as do the number and kind of allergens patients are allergic to—medical treatment of food allergies should be personalized or "tailor-made."[82] Such important advances notwithstanding, the fact remains that for people living with food allergies in 2022, there were few treatment options. Given that paucity of therapeutic alternatives, and the continued need for strict antigen avoidance, how is one to live meaningfully with life-threatening food allergies—when the next meal, could be one's last? To that important question, we now turn.

Conclusion: "To Live Is to Live with Death All the Time"
-or-
Learning to Surrender

"I depart as air, I shake my white locks at the runaway sun,
I effuse my flesh in eddies, and drift it in lacy jags.

I bequeath myself to the dirt to grow from the grass I love,
If you want me again look for me under your boot-soles."
—Walt Whitman, Leaves of Grass (1892)

"Be absolute for death...."
—William Shakespeare,
Measure for Measure (1604)

-◊-

I wrote this book in hopes of helping people living with food allergies—and their families, friends, teachers, and caregivers—to better understand the physiological and psychological effects of that disease. Food allergic people live every day in an uncomfortable proximity to illness and death, but at some point we all must face our own mortality, and that of those nearest and dearest to us. While hardly a cheering topic for those with extreme food allergies, or for parents worried about the survival of their children, what could be more important than cultivating healthy attitudes toward death and dying for people who confront their mortality every day, at every meal? Is it possible to transform the burden of food allergies into an opportunity for engagement with life on a more profound level?

While many of us would accept the proposition that stress can cause physical illness, did you know that feeling less fit in comparison to others may trim away years of your life, that what we read on food labels can affect the way our bodies process food, that placebo sugar pills can physically alter the body when one believes they will?[1] Did you realize that optimism, the tendency to believe that future expectations and goals will be met, has been linked by scientists to stronger immune systems, lower levels of inflammation and pain, greater psychological resiliency, reduced stress, longer lifespans, and other advantages?[2] By shifting our attitude about what many people would regard as the worst possible outcome of severe food allergies, i.e., sudden death, I contend that we may become more aware of the "minute particulars" of life: dawn light bursting through mountain trees, pink peonies at the peak of their flowering, black birds calling from a juniper tree, storm clouds lumbering through a blue sky, the scent of wet earth and leaves on a rainy autumn day, the radiant smile of a beloved child.

With that shift in perception, one that acquaints us with the truth of transience, we become more accepting of the movement of all things toward entropy (the second law of thermodynamics). As philosopher Jiddu Krishnamurti observes, "to live is to live with death all the time,"[3] yet most of us, including myself, tend to fear it. The term "death anxiety" refers to a cluster of phobias that uniquely assail human beings. Some of us fear the process of dying, some fear the loss of conscious awareness, some fear dying prematurely, some fear what will happen to the body, some fear for those "left behind," some fear punishment after death, some fear the unknown.[4] The fear of death is universal, and for all but the fortunate few, death involves pain and the loss of things that we hold dear.

Krishnamurti regarded fear as one of the greatest problems in life. "How can I," he asks, "who am a bundle of all these reactions, responses, memories, hopes, depressions, frustrations, who am the result of the movement of consciousness blocked," go beyond fear to find extraordinary joy in freedom from it?[5] Does a leaf that falls to the ground fear death, he asks? Does a bird live in fear of dying? No, because the bird is too preoccupied with living (catching insects, building a nest, singing, flying through the air) to be afraid. The bird lives from moment to moment, and simply meets death when it comes. Death frightens us because it means letting go of people, things, memories, and beliefs, and we tend to cling to what we've accumulated during our lifetimes, even though that attachment invites fear, pain, and suffering in a transient world.

People caught in physical or psychological fear tend to live lives full of confusion and conflict and to remain stuck in their own patterns of thinking. Is it possible, Krishnamurti asks, to recognize fear as a mental pattern that includes things like dread at the idea of losing your job, of not having enough money, of what your neighbors or coworkers think of you, of losing your position in society, of experiencing pain and disease, of not being loved, of not living up to the image others have built up about you? Can we recognize fear *as rooted in the non-acceptance of what is*, rather than trying to suppress it, control it, discipline it?[6] Might we learn to live without psychological fear by becoming acutely aware of sensations, of thought, of the body, and thereby to transcend the self and its preoccupations and discover true freedom?

-◊-

For food-allergic people like me, and those who develop other life-limiting ailments or disabilities, the contemplation of mortality lends meaning to life by charging it with intensity and authenticity. With unequivocal acceptance of the inevitability of our own demise, and of everyone and everything around us, we sanctify each moment. Strictly speaking, nothing and no one remains the same from one moment to the next, which is why religions of the East use metaphors of dreams, dust, clouds, and the passing of seasons to call attention to incessant change in the material world. Recognizing this transitoriness allows us to appreciate seemingly mundane things like the short blooming life of flowers or the buzz of cicadas who fall from the trees after singing their song. In Japan, Korea, and China, people celebrate the arrival of the cherry blossoms every spring, in part because they fall so quickly after their appearance. Sensitivity to the impermanence of all things makes us more appreciative of their flashing into the material world, and it elicits powerful emotions in us such as wistfulness at their passing.

Although most of us know intuitively that all life, including human life, is fragile and fleeting, we prefer not to linger too long or ponder too deeply on the truth of our own transience. But when we meet friends again after many years, we may notice how they've aged, and contemplate how we've changed too. Should we live long enough, we will know people who become ill unexpectedly, who weaken with age, who wither and die, it seems so suddenly. To suppress thoughts of our own demise, many of us keep busy with work, with raising families, with sensual pleasures, with entertaining diversions of various sorts, and so we drive from our conscious minds the fact that death is as inevitable as the alternation of day and night. Siddhartha Gautama, the Buddha, aimed to awaken people to the truth of transience not as a matter of doctrine, but as an incontrovertible fact. By learning to accept death as part of an unceasing transformation of the material world, we naturally ask, "how can I best live in the midst of it"?[7] By remembering that we shall die, we learn to live more fully.

Spiritual teachers and visionaries across time and culture have deployed their understanding of transience to cultivate great inner strength. Sen Rikyu, the founder of the Japanese tea ceremony, committed hara-kiri (ritual suicide by disembowelment) in 1591 at the order of Toyotomi Hideyoshi, a powerful sixteenth-century feudal lord and unifier of Japan. Sen Genshitsu, a descendent of Sen Rikyu, explains in his foreword to the *Book of Tea* (1906) by Okakura Kakuzo that the governing principle of the tea ceremony is elegantly simple: guests pass through a small garden of trees and shrubbery and enter the quiet space of a rustic tea room decorated with a single scroll and a few flowers tastefully arranged to create the atmosphere of an isolated retreat from the busy world. The preparation, consumption, and cleaning of tea and tea wares are executed with a quiet deliberateness that focuses attention on the present moment. Rikyu's tea ceremony may be conceived as a discipline in the "Art of Life" wherein the cultivation of mindfulness results in a greater appreciation of the ordinary aspects of everyday existence.[8]

Right before Rikyu took his own life at the order of Lord Hideyoshi for an unknown offense, he declared: "When I have this sword there is no Buddha and no Patriarchs."[9] Founder of the San Francisco Zen Center Shunryu Suzuki explains that before we were born, we were one with the universe, a state of consciousness referred to in Zen as "mind-only," "essence of mind," or "big mind." What Rikyu meant was that when we have the sword of big mind, there is no dualistic world. "This kind of imperturbable spirit was always present in Rikyu's tea ceremony," Suzuki observes. "He never did anything in just a dualistic way; he was ready to die in each moment. In ceremony after ceremony he died, and he renewed himself. This is the spirit of the tea ceremony."[10] In such a state of mind, writer François Cheng notes, ordinary experiences in daily life may interrupt otherwise automatic identification with thought and direct attention to the present moment. The direct experience of the fundamental nonduality of inner and outer (that "all things are one") instills a deep sense of purpose in life when one realizes that "a stream singing among the irises, an orange tree in the middle of a courtyard, [...] a dragonfly that lingers on a trembling reed, a lizard crossing a lichen-covered rock," and even the "sunset's rays highlighting a section of old wall," are entryways into presence.[11]

In the West, the Stoic philosopher Lucius Annaeus Seneca (Seneca the Younger) recommended that everyone "study death always," and through that investigation come to an understanding of the interconnectedness of all things. In his view, people must rehearse for death throughout their lives—and who better to understand that edifying practice than those living with food allergies who stare into the abyss with each food label, each restaurant meal, each invitation for dinner at someone's home? Seneca understood life as essentially a journey towards death, since we are dying every day from the moment we are born. He believed that we must accept death with unmitigated candor. That assertion was no mere platitude. When he received an order from the Emperor Nero to commit suicide after the discovery of a plot to stage a coup (though Seneca was likely innocent of the charge of complicity), Tacitus reports in the *Annals* (c. 109) that having learned to accept one's fate as divine will, Seneca embraced his wife, who attempted to die with him, one final time, and they "sundered with a dagger the arteries of their arms."[12] When Nero forbade her death, her bleeding was staunched. Seneca bled so slowly that he begged a close friend to concoct a poison for him, which he swallowed, though he eventually suffocated in a bath. According to Seneca's last wishes, his body was cremated without the usual funerary rites.[13]

The right to die, and to die well, remained essential to Seneca, whether that privilege meant accepting the biological processes of one's own decay with equanimity or choosing the time and method of one's exit. His writings on the subject are highly instructive in terms of how to live with death—and more meaningfully on account of it. In *Moral Epistles* (65 CE), Seneca writes to his close friend Lucilius and asks him to notice "the way that all things that seem to die are in fact only transformed." If one looks carefully, counsels the savant, one sees that "nothing in this cosmos is extinguished, but everything falls and rises by turns," like the seasons or the alternation of day and night. Thus, "the one who will return to the world should leave it."[14] Seneca suffered from asthma and depression his entire life, yet he regarded those attacks as a "rehearsal for death." In the "midst of suffocation," he concluded that death is merely nonexistence:

> I know what [death is] like. It will be the same after me as it was before me. If death holds any torment, then that torment must also have existed before we came forth into the light, but, back then, we felt nothing troubling. I ask

you, wouldn't you call it a very foolish thing if someone judges that a lamp is worse off after it's snuffed out than before it has been lighted? We too are snuffed out and lighted. In the time in between, we have sense and experience, before and after is true peace.[15]

Seneca also counseled moderation in all things, and he emphasized the necessity of contemplating "the brevity of one's life span, and its uncertainty. Whatever you undertake," he recommended to Lucilius, "cast your eyes on death."[16] If we take Seneca at his word, knowing that he "practiced what he preached," then those of us living with anaphylaxis might feel grateful for the opportunity to examine death more profoundly and thereby to live more deliberately. "Whoever doesn't want to die," Seneca asserted, "doesn't want to live."[17]

-◊-

While we may not control our destiny, we can choose our attitude toward it. Psychologist Viktor Frankl developed logotherapy, a therapeutic approach to finding meaning in life, after surviving imprisonment in four Nazi concentration camps and enduring the loss of his entire immediate family to them—save for one sister who had emigrated to Australia. He premised logotherapy on the notion that the primary motivational force in human beings is finding purpose by completing a work or task, by loving somebody or something fully, by the attitude adopted toward unavoidable suffering—rather than through power, money, or fame. Frankl witnessed far greater misery, suffering, and death in concentration camps than most of us experience in a lifetime. When he reflected on the prisoners whom he knew who survived the hunger, humiliation, fear, and injustice of the Holocaust, he discovered that religion and spirituality, memories of beloved persons, a macabre sense of humor, and a sensitivity to the healing power of nature lent meaning to people in otherwise intolerable situations.[18]

For those with food-induced anaphylaxis facing the specter of death every day, finding a way to accept the limitations that accompany that chronic condition is paramount to growing healthward. That possibility may elude younger children, but anyone old enough to read this book may begin the process of locating meaning in their suffering. The life stories of Seneca and Rikyu exemplify an ultimate human freedom that is essentially attitudinal. Daily life for prisoners in concentration camps made clear to Frankl that people always have a choice of action that preserves independence of mind and spiritual liberty—even under the most extreme forms of psychological and physical violence.

Conclusion

For Frankl, choosing how to respond to suffering represented one of the central tasks in life. He saw martyrs in the concentration camps walking through huts "giving away their last piece of bread. They may have been few in number, but they offer sufficient proof that everything can be taken from a man but one thing: the last of the human freedoms—to choose one's attitude in any given set of circumstances, to choose one's own way."[19]

Even when confronted with an unchangeable fate, an incurable disease like an inoperable cancer, we can still wrest meaning from life by becoming a witness to the ability to turn suffering into triumph. Some may find it in the beauty of nature or art; in a deed or a work that one creates; or by giving to a cause, serving others, or loving another person. The more one forgets oneself, the more human one becomes and the more one self-actualizes (as a side effect of transcendence). Frankl asserts "suffering ceases to be suffering at the moment it finds a meaning, such as the meaning of a sacrifice."[20] To illustrate that point, he recalls an elderly doctor who fell into a deep depression after the death of his wife. Instead of offering him advice, Frankl asked this man what would have happened had his wife survived him. "Oh," the doctor replied, "for her this would have been terrible; how she would have suffered!" Whereupon Frankl replied, "You see, Doctor, such a suffering has been spared her, and it was you who have spared her this suffering—to be sure, at the price that now you have to survive and mourn her."[21] Without a word, the doctor shook Frankl's hand and quietly left his office.

Even a helpless person in a desperate situation, facing a fate that cannot be altered, may "rise above himself, may grow beyond himself, and by doing so change himself."[22] That understanding came to Frankl when he realized that the deprivation, hardship, violence, murder, and indignity in the camps had enhanced his ability to help others. With the right attitude, the recognition of the truth of transience challenges us to make use of every moment to locate meaning, to find courage and dignity in suffering, and to act properly. As the philosopher Friedrich Nietzsche observed, "he who has a why to live for can bear with almost any how."[23] For that reason, logotherapy holds that mental and emotional disorders are often symptoms of an underlying sense of emptiness or meaninglessness and can be eliminated by finding one's own unique mission in life.[24] In other words, those of us living with anaphylactic food allergies have a unique opportunity to live more fully and deliberately.

-◊-

Conclusion: "To Live Is to Live with Death All the Time"

Internalizing the truth of transience and suffering is not to be a pessimist, but to be an activist (as in being disposed to take action or to effect change). Knowing that "all things must pass" does not mean relaxing vigilance needed to avoid food allergens, or to become careless when eating outside of the home. Rather, a clear perception of transience makes life more consequential. Through birth, each one of us miraculously becomes a warm breathing body, awake and alert, but eventually the spirit that animates that form departs, leaving behind a shell not unlike the abandoned exoskeleton of a cicada clinging to the bark of a tree. In her book, *Advice for Future Corpses* (2018), palliative-care nurse and Zen practitioner Sallie Tisdale encourages people to imagine their own death. She suggests that we visualize the time, the place, the season, the environment, and the complete details of our passing as a method for dealing with the deep-seated fear of self-extinction.[25]

Tisdale also appreciates that a dead body is the site of great activity. As consciousness departs during the process of death, the body takes on new life. Maggots reduce the weight of a carcass by 50 percent in a few weeks. Next, several waves of insects swarm the decomposing body and colonize it in a strict sequence. Blowflies and houseflies begin to blacken and soften it, and the meat on which maggots feed begins to liquify and run "like melting butter."[26] Fruit flies, drone flies, and others that prefer the liquids constitute the third wave, and toward the end, the cheese skipper appears and cleans the bones of the remnants of tendons and connective tissue. In that process, Tisdale observes the deep interconnectedness between the individual and the environment:

> I contemplate my ordinary, imperfect, beloved body. I contemplate the bodies of my beloveds: individual, singular, unique, irreplaceable people, their skin and eyes and mouths and hands. I consider their skin riddled and bristling with that seething billow of maggots. I consider the digestion of their eyes and the liquefaction of those hands (my hands, my eyes), the rending of flesh and muscle by beak and claw. The evolution of the person into a thing, into meat and wet carrion and eventually into a puddle, into new flies, into earth and root. What better vision of the fullness of birth and fullness of death than the maggot and carrion eater?

Because we're all going to die, Tisdale recommends making a death plan for our own peace of mind and for the sake of those nearest to us, who will be left to handle all manner of practical concerns. Decisions regarding what to do with the body (cremation or burial), any ceremonies we might desire, and the role that religion should play in such a gathering are relatively easy matters to outline.

Conclusion

For those of us with anaphylaxis, whom death may find unexpectedly at the most inopportune moment, visualizing an ideal passing, for example one surrounded by thoughtful caregivers who love us, with plenty of time to say our goodbyes, parse out any property we own, settle financial arrangements, and plan funerals seems somewhat unrealistic. Death via anaphylaxis may leave us with less than an hour of struggling for breath to come to grips with our impending demise. From a certain point of view, there's something positive about a quick death, but we should remember that teenager Karanbir Cheema died after ten days in intensive care.[27] So too, any benefit of passing quickly may prove cold comfort to those left behind. Rather than imagining an ideal death, as Tisdale suggests, I prefer to wonder if an accidental exposure will take me out in a matter of minutes, or whether my diligence in avoiding nuts will allow an unknown disease process related to old age to throw me into prolonged agony and pain. Time will tell, but in the latter case, I take some solace in the fact that one candy bar could end that suffering.

Tisdale's unusually open attitude about death springs from her dissection of cadavers in anatomy and physiology lab (where she became familiar with the odor of formaldehyde "and the faint leathery smell of the bodies,"), years as a palliative-care nurse, and her study of Zen Buddhism.[28] Those familiar with the central tenets of that tradition know that its teachings include the recognition of impermanence, the truth of suffering, and the doctrine of no-self (*anatman*). After reaching enlightenment under the Bodhi tree, the Buddha preached his first sermon, the Four Noble Truths. In it, he taught that human life is full of suffering, dissatisfaction, and unease—and that much of it stems from desire, craving, and attachment in a world where everything moves towards entropy. The Buddha preached that these mental defilements could be rooted out of the mind, and to accomplish that feat, he prescribed the Noble Eightfold Path, which included training in ethics (right action, right speech, right livelihood), concentration (right effort, right mindfulness, right concentration), and wisdom (right views and right intentions).

-◊-

When the Buddha experienced religious awakening, he realized that all beings have the same nature ("buddha nature") and potential for enlightenment. By seeing into the unitive and undifferentiated nature of reality that undergirds all phenomenon, we overcome the erroneous view of the self (the ego) as a separate and abiding entity. Shunryu

Suzuki confirms that "everything changes" is the basic truth for each existence:

> This teaching is also understood as the teaching of selflessness. Because each existence is in constant change, there is no abiding self. In fact, the self-nature of each existence is nothing but change itself, the self-nature of all existence. There is no special, separate self-nature for each existence. This is also called the teaching of Nirvana. When we realize the everlasting truth of "everything changes" and find our composure in it, we find ourselves in Nirvana.[29]

Nirvana, a term that means "to extinguish," involves a radically transformed state of consciousness in which greed and delusion are blown out like the flame of a candle. When one rids oneself of the erroneous notion that there exists a "separate self-nature for each existence," the personality is radically reconstituted so that negative mental states such as fear, anxiety, and doubt are replaced with a sense of deep peace, joy, compassion, and alert awareness.[30]

In asserting that there was no abiding "self" (*atman*), the Buddha did not mean that we don't exist here and now. Instead, he wanted to evoke the direct realization of oneself as fundamentally inseparable from nature—a single manifestation in a complex web of interconnectedness and interdependent arising from which a self cannot be extricated.[31] Through meditation and rational contemplation, the Buddhist practitioner seeks to know intuitively that the "self" is actually "no self" because it is a fleeting combination of elements (in Buddhist parlance five aggregates, eighteen constituents, six elements, six consciousnesses, and so forth). Indeed, when the Buddha enjoined a disciple to "train herself," that imperative indicated personhood, because as long as the aggregates abide, the person exists, and we say, "I walk, I think." To assert, however, that one's "self" is a "substantial personal identity, an enduring subject at the core of the aggregates, is mistaken."[32]

To illustrate the teaching of *anatman* (no-self), the Buddha employed the simile of the chariot. Just as a collection of parts arranged in a certain manner is conventionally understood as a chariot, when one starts to remove parts (wheels, harness, carriage, floorboards, axle, yoke), at a certain point it stops being a chariot.[33] So too, what most people take as "selfhood" is a temporary combination of elements over which we exercise very little control. To prove that point, the Buddha asked which of his disciples could demonstrate a level of power over the elements to prevent the body from aging or to subdue strong emotions by wishing them away.[34] Through meditation leading to insight,

Conclusion

Buddhists strive to break the misconception that a person is a permanent, unitary entity independent from its surroundings. The process of dispelling this misperception resembles peeling away the layers of an onion until nothing is left, or until just its absence ("emptiness") remains. As the influential second century philosopher Nagarjuna poetically explained:

> A person is not earth, not water,
> not fire, not wind, not space,
> not consciousness, and not all of them.
> What else could a person be?
>
> Just as a person is not real
> due to being a composite of six elements,
> so, too, is each of the elements
> not real due to being a composite.
>
> The aggregates are not the self, they are not in it;
> it is not in them, but without them, it is not;
> it is not mixed with the aggregates like fire and fuel.
> Therefore, how could the self exist?[35]

Because it is temporary, the self is empty of inherent existence. From this perspective, what we might call religion is simply a clear awareness that the individual is part of the nexus of life, and that meaning is found in relationship to that larger whole. In a real sense, the doctrine of "no-self" is simply the reassertion of the basic truth of transience.

So, how does this view of the self as "empty" help people with food allergies to live better lives? First, it shows us that our failure to accept the truth of impermanence causes suffering (when we cannot accept old age, sickness, and death). Second, while we may conceive of ourselves as separate entities, somehow different from the things we see around us, we are in fact part of a mutually dependent arising in which everything comes out of nothing at every moment, always fresh and new. What a miracle! Third, those of us living with life-threatening illnesses may use the beauty of nature to discover deeper meaning in existence by recognizing ourselves as change. We are that giant cloud that seems to have such solidity, white on top and dark at the bottom and filled with moisture, which is gradually blown apart by the wind until the last wisp disappears and merges with the sky.

When the Buddha extended the doctrine of no-self to all things, he meant that whatever we see in the world of matter (form) is transforming before our eyes, losing its equilibrium against a backdrop of exquisite balance (emptiness).[36] Form is emptiness, emptiness is form. There exists no duality, no separateness, no division between self and other. I am that which I see, I am expanded. "I am large, I contain multitudes," the poet and mystic Walt Whitman proclaimed.[37] When I recognize myself in the world of change, I begin to see more penetratingly because I've become sensitive to the ephemerality of all things. I begin, in the words of poet-painter William Blake, "To see the world in a grain of sand, / And Heaven in a wild flower, / Hold infinity in the palm of [my] hand / And eternity in an hour."[38] When one grasps this fact, not merely conceptually but by seeing deeply into it, one does not fear death quite so much anymore, whether from anaphylaxis today or another cause years from now. Besides, facing death head on, an essential skill for anyone living with anaphylaxis, teaches us to cultivate self-control, to put our own death (and the death of others) into a broader perspective, and to come to terms with the way things are—*not how we want them to be.*

-◊-

For readers who find it difficult to locate meaning in religious and spiritual teachings, reports of near-death experiences offer another opportunity to allay fears about death and dying by pointing towards something beyond the self. With increasing frequency, perhaps due to rising survival rates resulting from modern techniques of resuscitation, people who have survived life-threatening crises report extraordinary occurrences known as "near-death experiences." Although they contain universal elements that can be traced across culture and time, near-death experiences also contain specific individual, cultural, and religious elements that reflect their subjective nature. That is to say, while the content of near-death experiences and their effects on patients exhibit a universality worldwide, the vocabulary used to describe and to interpret them tends to be culturally bound and contain ethnocentric and localized phrasings that should be peeled away to reveal their "core elements."[39]

Near-death experiences occur in a variety of circumstances, including emergency situations where death seems unescapable like traffic accidents, and in cases of serious illness including anaphylactic or septic shock, cardiac arrest resulting in clinical death, electrocution, coma as a consequence of traumatic brain damage, attempted suicide, near-drowning or asphyxia, and apnea.[40] When near-death experiences occur in the terminal phase of an illness, they are called

Conclusion

"deathbed visions."[41] Some researchers believe that near-death and death experiences result from physiological changes in the brain, for instance when brain cells begin to die, while others posit that they stem from a psychological reaction to approaching death or from changes in consciousness (e.g., transcendence) in which perception, cognitive functioning, emotion, and sense of identity function independently of normal body-linked waking consciousness.[42] Most people reporting near-death experiences are psychologically healthy, though some show non-pathological signs of dissociation, a mental process of disconnection from one's thoughts, feelings, memories or sense of identity.[43]

Psychiatrist Raymond Moody, who coined the term "near-death experience" in his book *Life After Life* (1975), found evidence of near-death experiences from the ancient and medieval worlds in the Bible, Plato's *Dialogues*, the *Egyptian Book of the Dead*, and the *Tibetan Book of the Dead*—as well as in the folkloric traditions of Native Americans, South Pacific Islanders, and East and Central Asians.[44] His book ushered in the modern era of near-death research at a time when those experiences were deemed discrete phenomena. In subsequent decades, researchers and theoreticians around the world investigated and recorded near-death experiences, helping to move them from the realm of the fantastic and supernatural to the scientific and empirical. One leading researcher, psychiatrist Bruce Greyson, developed the Near-Death Experience Scale as a way to measure the depth of those experiences, which he defined as profound subjective events "with transcendental or mystical elements that many people experience on the threshold of death."[45]

Greyson asserts that near-death experiences contain common elements that may be classified as follows: (1) cognitive features of time distortion, thought acceleration, life review, and revelation; (2) affective features including feelings of peace, joy, cosmic unity, and encounters with light; (3) paranormal features of vivid senses, apparent extrasensory perception and precognitive visions, and out-of-body experiences; and (4) transcendental features of otherworldly encounters with mystical beings, visible spirits, and uncrossable borders.[46] Although research findings about near-death experiences are sometimes difficult to correlate, there are many reasons not to dismiss these experiences as "hallucinations." Once thought to be rare, near-death experiences occur in an estimated 17 percent of those who nearly die.[47] Individuals who report near-death experiences include those who were pronounced clinically dead but were subsequently resuscitated; individuals who, in the course of accidents or illnesses, feared that they were near death; and people who, dying, were able to describe their experiences in their final moments (in "deathbed visions").[48]

The most frequent features of near-death experiences include an overwhelming feeling of peace and of well-being (including freedom from pain), the impression of being located outside one's physical body, floating or drifting through darkness (sometimes described as a tunnel), becoming aware of a golden light, encountering and perhaps communicating with a "being of light," rapid successions of visual images of one's past, and experiencing another world of great beauty.[49] While some people having near-death experiences hear themselves declared dead and meet with deceased friends and relatives, not all near-death experiences are positive. Greyson classified rarer, distressing types of near-death experiences that phenomenologically resembled the blissful type, but were interpreted as terrifying: experiences of nonexistence or an eternal void and those with hellish imagery.[50] "Regardless of their cause or nature, transcendent near-death experiences often permanently alter" survivors' attitudes, beliefs, values, and behaviors.

The aftereffects of near-death experiences most frequently recounted include an increased spiritual awareness and concern for others, a lowered fear of death, a decline in overt materialism, and a lessened sense of competition. Near-death survivors tend to see themselves as integral parts of a benevolent and purposeful universe in which personal gain, particularly at others' expense, is no longer relevant—and they express a feeling of special importance or destiny and a strengthened belief in existence after death that they could not claim before.[51] Many people who have had near-death experiences convey a greater appreciation for life, a renewed sense of purpose, a greater confidence and flexibility in coping with life's vicissitudes, an increased emphasis on love and service, a decreased concern with securing the approval of others. One researcher, who used an instrument based on Frankl's logotherapy, found near-death experiencers reported positive changes in finding purpose and meaning in life, as well as in death acceptance.[52]

Among the negative aftereffects of near-death experiences revealed in the medical literature are the challenge of adapting to new values, attitudes, and interests; the difficulty of getting friends and family to understand new beliefs and behaviors; and the expectation that near-death experiencers had gained "superhuman patience and forgiveness or miraculous healing and prophetic powers" (and the expressed disappointment when that turned out not to be the case).[53] At times,

Conclusion

survivors of near-death experiences expressed frustration at returning unwillingly to the world, reluctancy to share those experiences for
fear of ridicule, and hesitancy to accept the conditions and limitations
of human relationships. In rare cases, the price of near-death experiences included "long-term depression, broken relationships, disrupted
careers, feelings of severe alienation, an inability to function in the
world, long years of struggling with the keen sense of altered reality."[54]

All of us are going to die, and most of us are afraid of death, often
because we don't know what lies beyond, what Hamlet calls "that undis-
covered country." Near-death experiences frequently report great calm,
loss of pain, leaving the body, and traveling through a tunnel into a
comforting and loving light. In the light, a light being, who may or may
not speak, offers the soul a life review. Some people pass through a sce-
nic landscape and encounter a border, which if crossed, results in death.
If one turns back instead, that person returns to life and may report
a near-death experience.[55] We often associate consciousness with the
brain, as a kind of byproduct of biology, but most near-death experiencers explain that their encounters happened while they were unconscious yet lucid.

-◊-

British scholar Mark Fox analyzed the testimonies of almost 100
survivors of near-death experiences in *Through the Valley of the Shadow
of Death* (2002). One mother from Missouri, who had a massive hemor-
rhage when she gave birth to her youngest child, lost consciousness and
found herself being sucked into a great whirling void in which she heard
a "tremendous vibrating hum."[56] Next, she was surrounded by a bril-
liant light and felt the presence of an invisible guide leading her onward.
Overwhelming sensations of love and warmth enveloped her, and she
wanted nothing more than to move closer to an even greater light that
"seemed to be radiating from somewhere just ahead."[57] At that moment,
a sudden sense of desolation overcame her, which was followed by
instructions to return to her family. After she recovered, remembrance
of her near-death experience infused her life with a novel sense of love
and well-being, and it alleviated her fear of death.

In the closing years of World War II, a 28-year-old wounded sol-
dier, recovering from injuries sustained in a tank explosion in Italy, suddenly found himself floating in the air and looking down from a point
just below the ceiling at his body on a hospital bed. As he pondered the
curiousness of such a perspective, he passed through the ceiling and

found himself moving in a tunnel towards "the sort of light you will get on a late spring, early summer morning just after sunrise."[58] Surrounded by that luminosity, he discerned a vast crowd of people in the distance on a sandy surface below. It came to him that he had died and that a reception committee—and subsequent judgment—awaited him. Another survivor, who also floated above his body, noted that "my conscience immediately weighed up my actions and judged me and what I did."[59] Others described relief from oppressive thoughts of dying, which were replaced by a strengthened belief in "an indestructible core in me and my fellow men."[60]

A few patients reported unpleasant near-death experiences that included fear, panic, out-of-body journeys, entry into a black void, sensing of an evil force, and entry into a hell-like environment. One man in cardiac arrest described descending deep into the earth where everything was gray and where he was overcome with anger and fear. A Christian, he intuitively understood that he was in hell, and he was lost. An evil being, perhaps the Devil, pulled him deeper down into the dark to suffer some unnamed punishment. In a panic, he sensed the presence of a divine being—Jesus Christ—who tried to save him. The man attempted to call out to the Savior, but could not, then he rushed again through the black void before awaking to doctors telling him that he would be okay.[61] Regardless of whether their near-death experiences were positive or negative, almost everyone claimed to be changed in a way that transformed their values and lives so that they might better benefit society.

Based on her work with modern mystics and near-death experiencers, theologian Judith Cressy believes that near-death experiences are part of a broader pattern of experiences that can occur in the context of death, as well as "childbirth, personal crisis, attending the death of another, or spontaneously."[62] Cressy notes parallels among reports of mystics and their "apparent dying," what we might call the death of the ego or self-transcendence, which is most often described symbolically.[63] Jesus, for instance, asserts in the Gospel of John: "unless one is born anew, he cannot see the kingdom of God" (John 3:3). Cressy finds similar accounts among Western mystics like Theresa of Avila who, after raptures accompanying contemplative prayer and meditation, recalled that:

> I thought I was being carried up to Heaven: the first persons I saw there were my mother and father, and such great things happened in so short a time.... I wish I could give a description of the least smallest part of what

Conclusion

I learned, but when I try to discover a way of doing so, I find it impossible, for while the light we see here and that other light are both light, there is no comparison between the two and the brightness of the sun seems quite dull if compared to the other.

After returning to ordinary consciousness, she was left with "little fear of death" of which formerly she had been "very much afraid."[64] Neuropsychiatrist Peter Fenwick and others have noted the importance of learning to surrender in order to facilitate a "good death."[65] This point seems especially relevant to those of us living with anaphylaxis and other life-threatening conditions. Knowing that we may unexpectedly be exposed to food allergens at any moment, especially when away from home, learning to practice non-attachment seems eminently sensible. According to some researchers, the inability to let go at the time of death may result in restlessness, which prevents a peaceful passing.[66] When one can surrender the idea of continued life and attachment to one's partner, one's pets, one's children, one's house, one's job, one's unfinished projects, then a smooth transition from life to death becomes possible.

-◊-

Speaking with children about the surrender of the ego is unlikely to prove meaningful until they grow older, but young people can be taught about death in a variety of ways, such as when a pet dies, or a dead bird is found in the backyard. Tenzin Gyatso, the Dalai Lama, believes that since we are all going to die, we might as well learn more about it! No place untouched by death exists, and forthright education on birth and death as a single process should be integrated effectively into school curricula.[67] An appreciation of transience can also spur us to work harder on our projects. For me, that has meant teaching with all my might and penning books which, hopefully, facilitate new insight. In such a way, one learns to avoid being overwhelmed by the superficial, the artificial, the imaginary, or the material. Only by "taming our minds," argues the Dalai Lama, "and fully facing the end of our lives," can we "fully live in the present moment."[68]

Peace activist Thich Nhat Hanh suggests that if there were no death, we could not even exist: "In every moment, many cells in your body have to die so that you can continue to live. Not only the cells of your body but all the feelings, perceptions and mental formations in the river of consciousness in you are born and die in every moment."[69] What the Buddha essentially taught, observes Hanh, is that there is no birth, no death, no coming, no going, no sameness, no difference, no permanent self, and no annihilation. In fact, when "we understand that we cannot be destroyed, we are liberated from fear. It is a great relief. We can enjoy life and appreciate it in a new way."[70] Or, as the inimitable comedian George Carlin put it on the Dick Cavett Show in 1992: "I am greater than the universe, lesser than the universe, and equal to the universe. And, these are the proofs: I'm greater than the universe because I can think about it and contain it within my head; I'm lesser than it, because that's obvious; and I'm equal to it because all the atoms in me are all the atoms that make up the universe, the same atoms identically. So, there I am, and what is to fear?"

From a transcendental point of view, phenomena are neither created nor destroyed, since they are in a constant state of manifesting. Thich Nhat Hanh believes that to grasp this point is to become free of fear, to become enlightened, and to perceive essential reality. Nirvana means living in a state of consciousness empty of all notions (even the concept of "nirvana" and "emptiness") and beyond ideas of permanence and impermanence.[71] Waves seem to form and disappear, but they are inextricably part of the ocean. As poet Khalil Gibran writes in *The Prophet* (1923): "what is it to die but to stand naked in the wind and melt into the sun? / And what is it to cease breathing, but to free the breath from its restless tides, that it may rise and expand and seek God unencumbered?"[72] Life and death are one, even as the river and ocean are one. The secret to death is found in the heart of life.

-◊-

Establishing a clear-eyed view of death in this concluding chapter seemed crucial, since death looms over everything for people with food-induced anaphylaxis, and a new view of mortality informed by transience allays the worst fears about one's own passing and that of others. To that end, if the foregoing discussion of religious and spiritual perspectives on death and dying, and of near-death and death-bed experiences, resonated with the reader, this project will have been worthwhile. During my research, I learned much about the allergic response; about current treatment options (and their limits); about children grappling with multiple food allergies and the concerns of their caregivers; about the sudden deaths of allergic people who could not get medical care quickly enough or did not carry epinephrine; about the psychology of fear and post-traumatic stress syndrome; about the importance of food in world cultures; about the difficulties of traveling overseas, accepting invitations to dinner, and eating in restaurants; about the decay of the body after death; and about the profound ways that our food allergies affect the people closest to us.

It would be wrong to suggest that through writing I have freed myself from fears of eating and dying from anaphylaxis. On the contrary, those fears persist: the night that a meal of frozen fish and canned beans inexplicably resulted in waking up in the middle of the night with a swollen tongue and lips; the biting peppercorn in salsa that caused burning and localized swelling in my mouth and prompted me to re-read ingredients and to look up both products online for undisclosed allergens; the mushroom and sausage pizza from a "safe" restaurant that caused waves of dread resulting from the realization that I could be dead in 45 minutes—which turned into a meditation on the transience of all life, on books unfinished, on classes untaught, on miles not driven, on people not met, on experiences lost. Even when eating at home, or in other safe environments, fearful thoughts still arise.

On the other hand, fear has a positive function in that it helps one to remain vigilant; it would be foolhardy to court anaphylaxis by eating with abandon or by not carrying medications. The arising of fearful thoughts may never cease, but one's attitude towards them can change. Who wants to live a life plagued by obsessive thoughts of death and dying with every meal, of repeatedly playing out imaginary scenarios involving contact with food allergens? Who wants to live everyday bogged down in memories of past encounters with tree nuts and speculations about future crises, instead of glorying in the here-now? In this respect, I've found a daily practice of seated meditation, and a study of Eastern philosophy and Western psychology, has helped me to become more sensitive to beauty in the world.[73]

Early this morning, I said goodbye to Savannah at the airport as she departed for Beijing, fully aware that we might never see each other again. Yet, I was filled with joy on the drive home at the beauty of the mist rolling off the hills around Ithaca at sunrise. Because of the food allergy, I am sometimes (though definitely not always) more present, patient, and accepting of my own and others' shortcomings, and while that affliction constrains my life in many ways, I remember the millions of people around the world suffering illnesses worse than my own. Rather than wallowing in self-pity, or cowering at home in fear, I'm learning to balance vigilance and adventurousness, safety and amplified precaution, work and presence at home. I can even be grateful for my food allergy, and for that attitude I thank singer Mandy Harvey, who writes in *Sensing the Rhythm: Finding My Voice in a World Without Sound* (2017) that her life has been so enriched by losing her hearing that, had she the option, she would choose to remain deaf. She has become "a better person," more sensitive "to other people's pain," more appreciative of "little blessings," and has gained a "better sense of what was truly important."[74]

Inspired by Michael Pollan's book *How to Change Your Mind* (2018), in which the author "trips" on several psychedelics, a colleague who teaches philosophy at a local college thought I should end this project by trying to eat a peanut—or two. I once tolerated peanuts and considered his suggestion for a sensational ending and even spent some time thinking about how such an attempt might look with medical care near at hand. In the end, such an act seemed foolhardy. While I regret giving up tolerance to peanuts (and coconut) after the last anaphylactic episode, I'm content to let the matter rest there, at least for now. After more than two decades of avoiding nuts at every meal, I recognize that as time passes my vigilance sometimes drops, as does that of people closest to me, and the next time that I accidently ingest trace amounts of an almond, pecan, or walnut may mean one final dance with anaphylaxis.

So, rather than eating a nut as a way of demonstrating that I overcame, if for an instant, a fear of food, I choose instead to focus on living more fully in the here-now, on accepting death as part of life, on striving to become more sensitive to beauty in the world. I hope this book gives readers the courage to live more fully on the razor's edge of the here-now—the only thing that truly exists—and through that experience to live a more meaningful life, whether short or unexpectedly long. As soon as each moment comes into being, it is already ending. Everything comes out of nothing at every moment. With this understanding, we affirm life by continually giving up the self and its trappings and merging with the infinite emptiness out of which all things arise—and return. *Om shanti, shanti, shanti.*

Chapter Notes

Chapter One

1. Susie Heller, "A Teen Died After Accidentally Eating a Chips Ahoy! Cookie Containing Peanuts." *Business Insider*, July 18, 2018, https://www.businessinsider.com/teen-died-after-eating-chips-ahoy-cookie-with-peanuts-2018-7.

2. Jackie Salo, "Mom's Heartbreaking Warning After Daughter with Allergies Dies from Eating a Cookie." *New York Post*, July 16, 2018. https://nypost.com/2018/07/16/moms-heartbreaking-warning-after-daughter-with-allergies-dies-from-eating-a-cookie/.

3. Heller, "A Teen Died After Accidentally Eating a Chips Ahoy! Cookie Containing Peanuts." *Business Insider*, July 18, 2018.

4. American Academy of Allergy Asthma and Immunology, *Allergy Facts and Figures*, https://www.aafa.org/allergy-facts/.

5. Stephen J. Galli, Mindy Tsai, and Adrian M. Piliponsky, "The Development of Allergic Inflammation." *Nature* 454.7203 (2008): 445–454. doi: 10.1038/nature07204.

6. Stephen J. Galli and Mindy Tsai, "IgE and Mast Cells in Allergic Disease." *Nature Medicine* 18.5 (2012): 693–704. doi: 10.1038/nm.2755.

7. Jill E. Winland-Brown and Brian Oscar Porter, "Respiratory Problems." in *Primary Care: Art and Science of Advanced Practice Nursing*, ed. Lynne Dunphy, Jill E. Winland-Brown, Brian Oscar Porter, Debera J. Thomas (Philadelphia, PA: F.A. Davis Company, 2015), 349.

8. Emily Ayshford, "Exploring Food Allergy Origins and Treatments." *Breakthroughs: Feinberg School of Medicine Research Office*, April 2019. https://www.feinberg.northwestern.edu/research/docs/newsletters/2019/april20191.pdf.

9. Antonella Cianferoni and Antonella Muraro, "Food-Induced Anaphylaxis." *Immunology and Allergy Clinics of North America* 32.1 (2012): 165–195. doi: 10.1016/j.iac.2011.10.002.

10. Stephen F. Kemp, Richard F. Lockey, and Estelle R. Simons, "Epinephrine: The Drug of Choice for Anaphylaxis—A Statement of the World Allergy Organization." *The World Allergy Organization Journal* Volume 1, Supplement 2 (2008): S18-S26. doi.org/10.1186/1939-4551-1-S2-S18.

11. Antonella Cianferoni and Antonella Muraro, "Food-Induced Anaphylaxis." *Immunology and Allergy Clinics of North America* 32.1 (2012): 165–195. doi: 10.1016/j.iac.2011.10.002.

12. Robert Adler, "The Clean Water Act: Has It Worked?" *Environmental Protection Agency Journal* 20.1–2 (1994): 11.

13. Ted Schettler, "Toxic Threats to Neurologic Development of Children." *Environmental Health Perspectives* 109. 6 (2001): 813–816.

14. U.S. Environmental Protection Agency, "Learn About Polychlorinated Biphenyls (PCBs)." https://www.epa.gov/pcbs/learn-about-polychlorinated-biphenyls-pcbs.

15. MaryJane K. Selgrade, et al., "Induction of Asthma and the Environment: What We Know and Need to Know." *Environmental Health Perspectives* 114.4 (2006): 615–619. doi: 10.1289/ehp.8376.

16. Charlotte Debras, et al.,

"Artificial Sweeteners and Cancer Risk: Results from the NutriNet-Santé Population-Based Cohort Study." *PLOS Medicine* 9.3 (2022): doi.org/10.1371/journal.pmed.1003950.

17. "Asthma." World Health Organization, https://www.who.int/newsroom/fact-sheets/detail/asthma.

18. Zave Chad, "Allergies in Children." *Paediatrics & Child Health.* 6.8 (2001): 555–566. doi: 10.1093/pch/6.8.555.

19. Julie Wang and Andrew Liu, "Food Allergies and Asthma." *Current Opinion in Allergy and Clinical Immunology* 11.3 (2011): 249–254.

20. Justin Greiwe, "Oral Food Challenges in Infants and Toddlers." in *Pediatric Allergy: Immunology and Allergy Clinics* (Philadelphia, PA: Elsevier Health Sciences, 2019), 482.

21. Susan Prescott and Katrina J. Allen, "Food Allergy: Riding the Second Wave of the Allergy Epidemic." *Pediatric Allergy and Immunology* 22.2 (2011): 155–160. doi.org/10.1111/j.1399–3038.2011.01145.x.

22. Aleena Banerji, et al., "Predictors of Hospital Admission for Food-Related Allergic Reactions That Present to the Emergency Department." *Annals of Allergy, Asthma & Immunology* 106.1 (2011): 42–48.

23. Brian Handwerk, "Why Do Humans Have Allergies? Parasite Infections May Be the Trigger." *Smithsonian Magazine*, October 29, 2015, https://www.smithsonianmag.com/science-nature/why-do-humans-have-allergies-parasite-infections-trigger-180957101/.

24. G.W. Wong, "Comparative Study of Food Allergy in Rural and Urban Chinese School Children." *Journal of Allergy and Clinical Immunology* 123.2 (2009): S32.

25. Catharine Paddock, "Hookworms and Allergies—Doctor Infects Himself for Experiment." *Medical News Today*, April 18, 2012, https://www.medicalnewstoday.com/articles/244238#1.

26. Alexandra Sifferlin, "Doctor Infects Himself with Hookworm for Health Experiment." *Time Magazine*, April 18, 2012, http://healthland.time.com/2012/04/18/doctor-infects-himself-with-parasites-for-health-experiment/.

27. Scott H. Sicherer, *Food Allergies: A Complete Guide for Eating When Your Life Depends on It* (Baltimore: Johns Hopkins University Press, 2013), 203.

28. Rose A. Cooper, Elizabeth A. Kensinger, and Maureen Ritchey, "Memories Fade: The Relationship Between Memory Vividness and Remembered Visual Salience." *Psychological Science* 30.5 (2019): 657–668.

29. Adrienne Rich, *Diving Into the Wreck: Poems 1971–1972* (New York: Norton, 1973), 22–24.

30. John Whiteclay Chambers, *The Oxford Companion to American Military History* (Oxford University Press, 2000), 134.

31. Kelly Tzoumis, *Toxic Chemicals in America: Controversies in Human and Environmental Health* (Santa Barbara, CA: ABC-CLIO, 2020), 200.

32. Sicherer, *Food Allergies*, 18.

33. "Prednisone." National Library of Medicine, Medline Plus, https://medlineplus.gov/druginfo/meds/a601102.html.

34. "Theophylline." National Library of Medicine, Medline Plus, https://medlineplus.gov/druginfo/meds/a681006.html.

35. Lilieana Stadler Mitrea, *Pharmacology* (Ontario: Natural Medicine Books, 2008), 47.

36. S. Christy Sadreameli, Emily P. Brigham, and Ajanta Patel, "The Surprising Reintroduction of Primatene Mist in the United States." *Annals of the American Thoracic Society* 16.10 (2019): 1234–1236.

37. Mary Stachyra Lopez, *Images of America: Centreville and Chantilly* (Charlestown, SC: Arcadia, 2014), 9.

38. "Senate Joint Resolution No. 24: Celebrating the Life of Paul Benjamin Ferrara." https://www.richmondsunlight.com/bill/2012/sj24/fulltext/.

39. "1981: Sus-Phrine: The Greatest Asthma Medicine Ever." *Asthma History Blogspot* http://asthmahistory.blogspot.

com/2017/03/1981-sus-phrin-greatest-asthma-medicine.html.

40. Laura Vozzella and Gregory S. Schneider, "Virginia General Assembly Approves Medicaid Expansion to 400,000 Low-income Residents." *Washington Post*, May 30, 2018.

41. Claude A. Frazier, *Coping with Food Allergy* (New York: Quadrangle, 1985), 128.

42. "Food Problems: Is It an Allergy or Intolerance." Cleveland Clinic, https://my.clevelandclinic.org/health/diseases/-10009-food-problems-is-it-an-allergy-or-intolerance.

43. Greg Winter, "F.D.A. Survey Finds Faulty Listings of Possible Food Allergens." *New York Times*, April 3, 2001.

44. Frazier, *Coping with Food Allergy*, 129.

45. Paul J. Hannaway, *Asthma—An Emerging Epidemic: A Manual for Patients with Asthma, Parents of Children with Asthma, Asthma Educators, Health-care Providers, School Nurses and Coaches* (Lighthouse Point, FLA: Lighthouse Press, 2002), 69.

46. Michael Gallagher, et al., "Strategies for Living with the Risk of Anaphylaxis in Adolescence: Qualitative Study of Young People and Their Parents." *Primary Care Respiratory Journal* 21.4 (2012): 392–397.

47. Luciana Kase Tanno, et al., "Asthma and Anaphylaxis." *Current Opinion in Allergy and Clinical Immunology* 19.5 (2019): 447–455. doi: 10.1097/ACI.0000000000000566.

48. Jennifer Tupper and Shaun Visser, "Anaphylaxis: A Review and Update." *Canadian Family Physician* 56.10 (2010): 1009–1011.

49. Sunday Clark, et al., "Frequency of U.S. Emergency Department Visits for Food-related Acute Allergic Reactions." *The Journal of Allergy and Clinical Immunology* 127.3 (2011): 682–683. doi: 10.1016/j.jaci.2010.10.040.

50. Chungchan Gao, *African Americans in the Reconstruction Era* (New York: Routledge, 2016), 267.

51. Benjamin Campbell, *Richmond's Unhealed History* (Richmond, VA: Brandylane Publishers, 2012), 134–135.

Chapter Two

1. Stephen Addiss, *The Art of Haiku: Its History Through Poems and Paintings by Japanese Masters* (Boulder, CO: Shambhala, 2012), 24.

2. Paul Ham, *Hiroshima Nagasaki: The Real Story of the Atomic Bombings and Their Aftermath* (New York: St. Martin's, 2014), 152.

3. Jennifer Tupper and Shaun Visser, "Anaphylaxis: A Review and Update." *Canadian Family Physician* 56.10 (2010): 1009–1011.

4. Stephen E. Lapinsky, "Endotracheal Intubation in the ICU." *Critical Care* 19.1 (2015): 258. doi: 10.1186/s13054–015–0964-z

5. Paris Achen, "Turkey: Hazelnut Capital of the World." *Capital Press*, September 3, 2019, https://www.capitalpress.com/ag_sectors/orchards_nuts_vines/turkey-hazelnut-capital-of-the-world/article_2b403308-ce5e-11e9-bff9-1b26383e83a6.html.

6. "The Food Allergy Epidemic." *FARE*, https://www.foodallergy.org/resources/facts-and-statistics.

7. "Food Allergies." *CDC Healthy Schools*, https://www.cdc.gov/healthyschools/foodallergies/index.htm.

8. Zbigniew Bartuzi, et al., "The Diagnosis and Management of Food Allergies." *Advances in Dermatology and Allergology* 34.5 (2017): 391–404. doi: 10.5114/ada.2017.71104.

9. Alexander S. Zhovmer, "Novel and Emerging Therapies for Food Allergy." United States Food and Drug Administration, https://www.fda.gov/vaccines-blood-biologics/-biologics-research-projects/novel-and-emerging-therapies-food-allergy.

10. "Food Allergies." United States Food and Drug Administration, https://www.fda.gov/food/food-labeling-nutrition/food-allergies.

Chapter Three

1. Harry R. Moody, *Abundance of Life: Human Development Policies for an Aging Society* (New York: Columbia University Press, 1988), 79.

2. Djin Gie Liem and Catherine Georgina Russell, "The Influence of Taste Liking on the Consumption of Nutrient Rich and Nutrient Poor Foods." *Frontiers in Nutrition*, November 15, 2019, doi.org/10.3389/fnut.2019.00174.

3. Sreedhar Reddy and M. Anitha, "Culture and Its Influence on Nutrition and Oral Health," *Biomedical & Pharmacology Journal* 8 (2015): 613–620, doi.org/10.13005/bpj/757.

4. Gillian Crowther, *Eating Culture: An Anthropological Guide to Food* (University of Toronto Press, 2013), 15.

5. Crowther, *Eating Culture*, 10.

6. Crowther, *Eating Culture*, 152.

7. Lisa M. Bartnikas, et al., "Impact of School Peanut-Free Policies on Epinephrine Administration." *Journal of Allergy and Clinical Immunology* 140.2 (2017): 465–473. doi: 10.1016/j.jaci.2017.01.040.

8. Gwen Smith, "Sabrina's Law: The Girl and the Food Allergy Law." *Allergic Living*, July 2, 2010, https://www.allergicliving.com/2010/07/02/sabrinas-law-the-girl-and-the-allergy-law/.

9. Jo C. Phelan, et al., "Stigma, Status, and Population Health." *Social Science and Medicine* 103 (2014): 15–23. doi: 10.1016/j.socscimed.2013.10.004.

10. Jeremy C. Kane, et al., "A Scoping Review of Health-related Stigma Outcomes for High-burden Diseases in Low- and Middle-income Countries." *BMC Medicine* 17 (2019): 17. doi: 10.1186/s12916–019–1250–8.

11. Heinrich Troster, "Disclose or Conceal? Strategies of Information Management in Persons with Epilepsy." *Epilepsiu* 38.11 (1997): 1227–1237, doi.org/10.1111/j.1528–1157.1997.tb01221.x.

12. Jennifer Dean, et al., "Disclosing Food Allergy Status in Schools: Health-Related Stigma Among School Children in Ontario." *Health and Social Care in the Community* 24.5 (2016): e43-e52. doi.org/10.1111/hsc.12244.

13. Dean, et al., "Disclosing Food Allergy Status in Schools: Health-Related Stigma Among School Children in Ontario." *Health and Social Care in the Community* 24.5 (2016): e43-e52.

14. Margaret A. Sampson, et al., "Risk-taking and Coping Strategies of Adolescents and Young Adults with Food Allergy." *The Journal of Allergy and Clinical Immunology* 117.6 (2006): 1440–1445.

15. James Poniewozik, "Anthony Bourdain: The Man Who Ate the World." *New York Times*, June 8, 2018, https://www.nytimes.com/2018/06/08/arts/television/bourdain-death.html.

16. Carrie L. Masia, et al., "Peanut Allergy in Children: Psychological Issues and Clinical Considerations." *Education and Treatment of Children* 21.4 (1998): 514–531.

17. Patrick Bennett, "Developing an Adult Food Allergy Is a Life-Changer." *Allergic Living*, https://www.allergicliving.com/2016/01/19/when-allergy-strikes-an-adult/.

18. Gregor Hasler, et al., "Asthma and Panic in Young Adults: A 20-Year Prospective Community Study." *American Journal of Respiratory and Critical Care Medicine* 171.11 (2005): 1224–1230.

doi: 10.1164/rccm.200412–1669OC.

19. Lars Lange, "Quality of Life in the Setting of Anaphylaxis and Food Allergy." *Allergo Journal International* 23.7 (2014): 252–260. doi: 10.1007/s40629–014–0029-x.

20. Perri Klass, "Life-Threatening Allergic Reactions Rising in Children." *New York Times*, April 9, 2018, https://www.nytimes.com/2018/04/09/well/family/life-threatening-allergic-reactions-rising-in-children.html.

21. Youngsoo Lee, et al., "A Prospective Observation of Psychological Distress in Patients with Anaphylaxis." *Allergy, Asthma & Immunology Research* 12.3 (2020): 496–506, doi: 10.4168/aair.2020.12.3.496.

22. Man Cheung Chung, et al., "Trauma Exposure Characteristics, Past Traumatic Life Events, Coping Strategies, Posttraumatic Stress Disorder, and Psychiatric Comorbidity Among People with Anaphylactic Shock Experience." *Comprehensive Psychiatry* 52.4 (2011): 394–404.

23. Youngsoo Lee, et al., "A Prospective Observation of Psychological Distress in Patients with Anaphylaxis." 12.3

(2020): 496–506, doi: 10.4168/aair.2020. 12.3.496.

24. Jennifer Van Evra, "When Allergies Lead to Fear of Food." *Allergic Living*, July 2, 2010, https://www.allergicliving. com/2010/07/02/food-allergy-fear-of-food/.

25. Van Evra, "When Allergies Lead to Fear of Food." *Allergic Living*, July 2, 2010.

26. Van Evra, "When Allergies Lead to Fear of Food." *Allergic Living*, July 2, 2010.

27. Van Evra, "When Allergies Lead to Fear of Food." *Allergic Living*, July 2, 2010.

28. Van Evra, "When Allergies Lead to Fear of Food." *Allergic Living*, July 2, 2010.

29. Jan Plamper and Benjamin Lazier, *Fear: Across the Disciplines* (University of Pittsburg Press, 2012), 45.

30. Arash Javanbakht and Linda Saab, "What Happens in the Brain When We Feel Fear, and Why Some of Us Just Can't Get Enough of It." *Smithsonian Magazine*, October 27, 2017, https://www.smithsonianmag.com/-science-nature/what-happens-brain-feel-fear-180966992/.

31. Plamper and Lazier, *Fear: Across the Disciplines*, 38.

32. Plamper and Lazier, *Fear: Across the Disciplines*, 46.

33. Plamper and Lazier, *Fear: Across the Disciplines*, 50.

34. "Anxiety Disorders." National Institute of Mental Health, https://www.nimh.nih.gov/health/topics/anxiety-disorders.

35. Don H. Hockenbury and Sandra E. Hockenbury, *Psychology* (New York: Worth Publishers, 2003), G-10.

36. Josephine Howard-Ruben, "The Dangers of Flying While Allergic." *Scientific* American, February 13, 2019, https://blogs.scientificamerican.com/observations/the-dangers-of-flying-while-allergic/.

37. Adam Friedlander, "2020: Undeclared Allergens Continue to Be the Leading Cause of U.S. Food Recalls" *The Food Industry Association*, Nov 19, 2020, https://www.fmi.org/blog/view/fmi-blog/2020/11/19/2020-undeclared-allergens-continue-to-be-the-leading-cause-of-u.s.-food-recalls.

38. Robyn Eckhardt, *Istanbul and Beyond: Exploring the Diverse Cuisines of Turkey* (New York: Houghton Mifflin Harcourt, 2017), 31.

39. Holly Hazlett-Stevens, *Psychological Approaches to Generalized Anxiety Disorder: A Clinician's Guide to Assessment and Treatment* (New York: Springer, 2008), 147.

40. Jeffrey Alan Gray, *The Psychology of Fear and Stress* (Cambridge University Press, 1987), 208.

41. Phil Lieberman, "Reactions to Peanut During Air Travel: Can Anaphylaxis Be Due to Inhalation?" *American Academy of Allergy, Asthma & Immunology*, https://www.aaaai.org/allergist-resources/-ask-the-expert/answers/old-ask-the-experts/peanut-air-travel.

Chapter Four

1. Harvey L. Leo and Noreen M. Clark, "Managing Children with Food Allergies in Childcare and School." *Current Allergy & Asthma Reports* 7 (2007): 187–191, doi: 10.1007/s11882-007-0020-4.

2. Carrie L. Masia, et al., "Peanut Allergy in Children: Psychological Issues and Clinical Considerations." *Education and Treatment of Children* 21.4 (1998): 514–531.

3. Perla A. Vargas, "Developing a Food Allergy Curriculum for Parents." *Pediatric Allergy & Immunology* 22.6 (2011): 575–582, doi: 10.1111/j.1399-3038.2011.01152.x.

4. Scott Sicherer, et al., "The U.S. Peanut and Tree Nut Allergy Registry: Characteristics of Reactions in Schools and Day Care." *The Journal of Pediatrics* 138.4 (2001): 560–565, doi: 10.1067/mpd.2001.111821.

5. Scott H. Sicherer, et al., "Management of Food Allergy in the School Setting." *Pediatrics* 126.6 (2010): 1232–1239, doi.org/10.1542/peds.2010–2575.

6. Hugh A. Sampson, "Food Allergy: Past, Present and Future." *Allergology International* 65.4 (2016): 363–369, doi.org/10.1016/j.alit.2016.08.006.

7. D'Andra Millsap Shu, "Food Allergy Bullying as Disability Harassment:

Holding Schools Accountable," *University of Colorado Law Review*, February 1, 2021, https://lawreview.colorado.edu/printed/food-allergy-bullying-as-disability-harassment-holding-schools-accountable/.

8. New York State Department of Health, "Making the Difference: Caring for Students with Life-Threatening Allergies." https://www.health.ny.gov/professionals/protocols_and_guidelines/docs/caring_for_students_with_life_threatening_allergies.pdf.

9. New York State Department of Health, "Making the Difference: Caring for Students with Life-Threatening Allergies." https://www.health.ny.gov/professionals/protocols_and_guidelines/docs/caring_for_students_with_life_threatening_allergies.pdf.

10. Susan Weissman, *Feeding Eden: The Trials and Triumphs of a Food Allergy Family* (New York: Sterling Publishing, 2012), 2.

11. Weissman, *Feeding Eden*, 1.

12. Weissman, *Feeding Eden*, 3.

13. Weissman, *Feeding Eden*, 5.

14. Bright Nwaru, et al., "Idiopathic Anaphylaxis." *Current Treatment Options in Allergy* 4.3 (2017): 312–319, doi: 10.1007/s40521–017–0136–2.

15. Weissman, *Feeding Eden*, 9.

16. Weissman, *Feeding Eden*, 9.

17. Lisa Cipriano Collins, *Caring for Your Child with Severe Food Allergies* (New York: Wiley, 1999), 4.

18. Collins, *Caring for Your Child with Severe Food Allergies*, 5.

19. Collins, *Caring for Your Child with Severe Food Allergies*, 5.

20. Collins, *Caring for Your Child with Severe Food Allergies*, 6.

21. Carrie L. Masia, et al., "Peanut Allergy in Children: Psychological Issues and Clinical Considerations." *Education and Treatment of Children* 21.4 (1998): 514–531.

22. Gina Clowes, "Siblings and Food Allergies: Don't Overlook Needs of Your Non-Allergic Child," *Allergic Living*, https://www.allergicliving.com/2018/09/19/siblings-and-food-allergies-dont-overlook-the-needs-of-your-non-allergic-child/.

23. A.J. Cummings, "The Psychosocial Impact of Food Allergy and Food Hypersensitivity in Children, Adolescents and Their Families: A Review." *Allergy: The European Journal of Allergy and Critical Immunology* 65 (2010): 933–945, doi.org/10.1111/j.1398–9995.2010.02342.x.

24. Collins, *Caring for Your Child with Severe Food Allergies*, 59–60.

25. Collins, *Caring for Your Child with Severe Food Allergies*, 38.

26. D'Andra Millsap Shu, "Food Allergy Bullying as Disability Harassment: Holding Schools Accountable." *University of Colorado Law Review*, February 1, 2021, https://lawreview.colorado.edu/printed/food-allergy-bullying-as-disability-harassment-holding-schools-accountable/.

27. Marie-Louise Stjerna, "Food, Risk and Place: Agency and Negotiations of Young People with Food Allergy." *Sociology of Health & Illness* 37.2 (2015): 284–297, doi.org/10.1111/1467–9566.12215.

28. Marie-Louise Stjerna, "Food, Risk and Place: Agency and Negotiations of Young People with Food Allergy." *Sociology of Health & Illness* 37.2 (2015): 284–297.

29. A.J. Cummings, "The Psychosocial Impact of Food Allergy and Food Hypersensitivity in Children, Adolescents And Their Families: A Review." *Allergy: The European Journal of Allergy and Critical Immunology* 65 (2010): 933–945, doi.org/10.1111/j.1398–9995.2010.02342.x.

30. Jeremy K. Fox and Carrie Masia Warner, "Food Allergy and Social Anxiety in a Community Sample of Adolescents." *Children's Health Care* 46.1 (2017): 93–107, http://dx.doi.org/10.1080/02739615.2015.1124773.

31. Marie-Louise Stjerna, "Food, Risk and Place: Agency and Negotiations of Young People with Food Allergy." *Sociology of Health & Illness* 37.2 (2015): 284–297, doi.org/10.1111/1467–9566.12215.

32. Marie-Louise Stjerna, "Food, Risk and Place: Agency and Negotiations of Young People with Food Allergy." *Sociology of Health & Illness* 37.2 (2015): 284–297.

33. Kristina L. Newman, "Beliefs About Food Allergies in Adolescents

Aged 11–19 Years: A Systematic Review." *Clinical & Translational Allergy* 12.4 (2022): e12142, doi: 10.1002/clt2.12142.

34. Linda J. Herbert and Lynnda M. Dahlquist, "Perceived History of Anaphylaxis and Parental Overprotection, Autonomy, Anxiety, and Depression in Food Allergic Young Adults." *Journal of Clinical Psychology in Medical Settings* 15 (2008): 261–269, doi.org/10.1007/s10880–008–9130-y.

35. Jay A. Lieberman, et al., "The Global Burden of Illness of Peanut Allergy: A Comprehensive Literature Review." *Allergy: The European Journal of Allergy and Critical Immunology* 76 (2021): 1367–1384, doi.org/10.1111/all.14666.

36. Marie-Louise Stjerna, "Food, Risk and Place: Agency and Negotiations of Young People with Food Allergy." *Sociology of Health & Illness* 37.2 (2015): 284–297, doi.org/10.1111/1467–9566.12215.

37. Marie-Louise Stjerna, "Food, Risk and Place: Agency and Negotiations of Young People with Food Allergy." *Sociology of Health & Illness* 37.2 (2015): 284–297.

38. Marie-Louise Stjerna, "Food, Risk and Place: Agency and Negotiations of Young People with Food Allergy." *Sociology of Health & Illness* 37.2 (2015): 284–297.

39. Marie-Louise Stjerna, "Food, Risk and Place: Agency and Negotiations of Young People with Food Allergy." *Sociology of Health & Illness* 37.2 (2015): 284–297.

40. Jay A. Lieberman, et al., "Bullying Among Pediatric Patients with Food Allergy." Annals of *Allergy, Asthma & Immunology* 105.4 (2010): 282–286, doi.org/10.1016/j.anai.2010.07.011

41. Kimberly Holland, "The Furor Over the Peter Rabbit 'Food Allergy Scene,'" *Healthline*, February 23, 2018.

42. Kimberly Holland, "The Furor Over the Peter Rabbit 'Food Allergy Scene,'" *Healthline*, February 23, 2018.

43. Roni Caryn Rabin, "In Allergy Bullying, Food Can Hurt." *New York Times*, February 15, 2018, https://www.nytimes.com/2018/02/15/well/family/in-allergy-bullying-food-can-hurt.html.

44. Lisa O'Carroll, "Boy Dies After Allergic Reaction to Cheese Allegedly Forced on Him." *The Guardian*, July 11, 2017, https://www.theguardian.com/uk-news/2017/jul/11/karanbir-cheema-dies-allergic-reaction-cheese-allegedly-forced-on-him.

45. Barbara Davies, "I Can't Forgive the Cruel Bully Who Killed My Son." *Daily Mail*, May 10, 2019, https://www.dailymail.co.uk/news/article-7016559/-Mother-boy-13-died-pupil-threw-cheese-says-forgive-bully.html

46. Caroline Connell, "Food Allergy Bullying at School is on the Rise." *Allergic Living*, September 17, 2012, https://www.allergicliving.com/2012/09/17/-food-allergy-bullying-on-the-rise/.

47. Antonella Muraro, et al., "Comparison of Bullying of Food-allergic Versus Healthy School children in Italy." *Annals of Allergy, Asthma & Immunology* 105.4 (2010): 282–286, doi.org/10.1016/j.anai.2010.07.011.

48. Tove Danovich, "Parents, Schools Step Up Efforts to Combat Food-Allergy Bullying." *National Public Radio*, June 5, 2018, https://www.npr.org/sections/thesalt/2018/06/05/613933607/parents-schools-step-up-efforts-to-combat-food-allergy-bullying.

49. Rachel Annunziato, et al., "Longitudinal Evaluation of Food Allergy–Related Bullying." The *Journal of Allergy and Clinical Immunology* 2.5 (2014): 639–641, doi.org/10.1016/j.jaip.2014.05.001.

50. D'Andra Millsap Shu, "Food Allergy Bullying as Disability Harassment: Holding Schools Accountable," *University of Colorado Law Review*, February 1, 2021, https://lawreview.colorado.edu/printed/food-allergy-bullying-as-disability-harassment-holding-schools-accountable/.

51. Marwa Eltagouri, "Three Teens Charged with Knowingly Exposing Allergic Classmate to Pineapple." *Washington Post*, Jan 27, 2018, https://www.washingtonpost.com/news/education/wp/2018/01/26/3-teens-charged-with-knowingly-exposing-allergic-classmate-to-pineapple-she-was-hospitalized/.

52. Mariam Matti, "Michigan Student

Pleads Guilty in Peanut Butter Face-Smearing Case." *Allergic Living*, September 6, 2017, https://www.allergicliving.com/2017/09/06/michigan-student-pleads-guilty-in-peanut-butter-face-smearing-case/.

53. Jason Silverstein, "Panera Put Peanut Butter on Girl's Sandwich Despite Severe Allergy, Leading to Hospitalization, Lawsuit Says." *New York Daily News*, June 6, 2016, https://www.nydailynews.com/news/national/panera-put-peanut-butter-girl-sandwich-allergy-suit-article-1.2663106.

54. Cleveland Clinic, "How to Help Your Child Deal with Food Allergy Bullying." November 5, 2020, https://health.clevelandclinic.org/is-your-child-being-bullied-because-of-food-allergies-5-tips/.

55. Harshna Mehta, "Growth and Nutritional Concerns in Children with Food Allergy." *Current Opinion in Allergy and Clinical Immunology* 13.3 (2013): 275–279, doi: 10.1097/ACI.0b013e328360949d

56. Bethany Bray, "Supporting Clients Through the Anxiety and Exhaustion of Food Allergies." *Counseling Today*, November 27, 2018, https://ct.counseling.org/category/counseling-today/.

57. Jessica Taylor and Chrystal Lewis, "Counseling Adults With Food Allergies After an Anaphylactic Reaction: An Application of Emotion-Focused Therapy." *Journal of Mental Health Counseling* 40.1 (2018): 14–25, doi.org/10.17744/mehc.40.1.02.

58. Rose Kivi, "Acute Stress Disorder." *Healthline*, September 29, 2018, https://www.healthline.com/health/acute-stress-disorder.

59. Anushka Pai, et al., "Posttraumatic Stress Disorder in the DSM-5: Controversy, Change, and Conceptual Considerations." *Behavioral Science* 7.1 (2017): 1–7, doi: 10.3390/bs7010007.

60. U.S. Food & Drug Administration, "Food Allergies." https://www.fda.gov/food/food-labeling-nutrition/food-allergies.

61. Mandy Harvey, *Sensing the Rhythm: Finding My Voice in a World Without Sound* (New York: Howard Books, 2017), 162.

62. Scott H. Sicherer, *Food Allergies: A Complete Guide for Eating When Your Life Depends on It* (Baltimore, MD: Johns Hopkins University Press, 2017), 254.

63. U.S. Food & Drug Administration, "FDA Approves First Drug for Treatment of Peanut Allergy for Children." https://www.fda.gov/news-events/press-announcements/fda-approves-first-drug-treatment-peanut-allergy-children.

64. Roni Caryn Rabin "For Children with Peanut Allergies, F.D.A. Experts Recommend a New Treatment." *New York Times*, Sept. 13, 2019, https://www.nytimes.com/2019/09/13/health/peanut-allergy-children.html

65. William Moote and Harold Kim, "Allergen-specific Immunotherapy." *Allergy, Asthma & Clinical Immunology* 7 (2011): 1–7, doi: 10.1186/s13223-018-0282-5.

66. Wong Yu, et al., "Food Allergy: Immune Mechanisms, Diagnosis and Immunotherapy." *Nature Reviews Immunology* 16.12 (2016): 751–765, doi: 10.1038/nri.2016.111.

67. Jeanne Lomas and Kirsi Järvinen, "Managing Nut-induced Anaphylaxis: Challenges and Solutions." *Journal of Asthma and Allergy* 8 (2015): 115–123, doi: 10.2147/JAA.S89121.

68. T. Mousallem and A.W. Burks, "Immunology in the Clinic Review Series; Focus on Allergies: Immunotherapy for Food Allergy." *Clinical and Experimental Immunology* 167.1 (2012): 26–31, doi: 10.1111/j.1365-2249.2011.04499.x.

69. Wendy Mondello, "Girl with Milk Allergy Dies of Severe Reaction Related to Desensitization." *Allergic Living*, December 20, 2021, https://www.allergicliving.com/2021/12/20/girl-with-milk-allergy-dies-of-severe-reaction-related-to-desensitization/.

70. Jørgen Nedergaard Larsen, et al., "Allergy Immunotherapy: The Future of Allergy Treatment." *Drug Discovery Today* 21.1 (2016): 26–37, doi.org/10.1016/j.drudis.2015.07.010.

71. David M. Fleischer, et al., "Effect of Epicutaneous Immunotherapy vs Placebo on Reaction to Peanut Protein Ingestion Among Children with Peanut Allergy." *Journal of the American*

Medical Association 321.10 (2019): 946–955, doi: 10.1001/jama.2019.1113.

72. T. Mousallem and A.W. Burks, "Immunology in the Clinic Review Series; Focus on Allergies: Immunotherapy for Food Allergy." *Clinical and Experimental Immunology* 167.1 (2012): 26–31.

73. Brian P. Vickery, "Sustained Unresponsiveness to Peanut in Subjects Who Have Completed Peanut Oral Immunotherapy." *The Journal of Allergy and Clinical Immunology* 133.2 (2014): 468–75, doi: 10.1016/j.jaci.2013.11.007.

74. Howe, Lauren, et al. "Changing Patient Mindsets About Non–Life-Threatening Symptoms During Oral Immunotherapy: A Randomized Clinical Trial." *The Journal of Allergy and Clinical Immunology* 7.5 (2019): 1550–1559, doi: 10.1016/j.jaip.2019.01.022.

75. "Aravax Takes a Step Closer to Developing a Peanut Allergy Vaccine." *Pharmaceutical Technology*, March 9, 2019, https://www.pharmaceutical-technology.com/comment/aravax-takes-a-step-closer-to-developing-a-peanut-allergy-vaccine/.

76. Elizabeth Feuille and Anna Nowak-Wegrzyn, "Allergen-Specific Immunotherapies for Food Allergy." *Allergy, Asthma & Immunology Research* 10.3 (2018): 189–206, doi: 10.4168/aair.2018.10.3.189.

77. Arnau Navinés-Ferrer, et al., "IgE-Related Chronic Diseases and Anti-IgE-Based Treatments." *Journal of Immunology Research* (2016): 1–12, doi: 10.1155/2016/8163803.

78. Khui Hung Lee, et al., "The Gut Microbiota, Environmental Factors, and Links to the Development of Food Allergy." *Clinical and Molecular Allergy* 18.5 (2020): 1–11, doi.org/10.1186/s12948-020-00120-x

79. Gagné, Claire. "Dr. Li and Her Chinese Herbal Remedies." *Allergic Living*, December 15, 2015. https://www.allergicliving.com/2015/12/15/dr-li-and-her-chinese-herbal-remedies/.

80. Claire Gagne, "Dr. Li and Her Chinese Herbal Remedies." *Allergic Living*, December 15, 2015.

81. Lauren Lisann, et al., "Successful Prevention of Extremely Frequent and Severe Food Anaphylaxis In Three Children By Combined Traditional Chinese Medicine Therapy." *Allergy, Asthma & Clinical Immunology* 10 (2014): 1–11, doi. org/10.1186/s13223–014–0066–5.

82. Naomi Kondo, et al., "Medical Treatment of Food Allergies Should be Personalized." *Personalized Medicine Universe* 4 (2015): 73–75, doi. org/10.1016/j.pmu.2015.03.005.

Conclusion

1. Esther Landhuis, "Could Your Mindset Affect How Well a Treatment Works?" *National Public Radio*, March 1, 2019, https://www.npr.org/sections/-health-shots/2019/03/01/699399504/-could-your-mindset-affect-how-well-a-treatment-works.

2. "Think Positive For Better Health: Changing Negative Thought Patterns to Positive May Boost Physical and Mental Health as Well as Lifespan," *Mind, Mood & Memory* 7.7 (2011): 3.

3. Jiddu Krishnamurti, "3rd Question & Answer Meeting." Switzerland—July 26, 1983, https://jkrishnamurti.org/content/3rd-question-answer-meeting-14.

4. James Gire, "How Death Imitates Life: Cultural Influences on Conceptions of Death and Dying." *Online Readings in Psychology and Culture* 6.2 (2014): 1–22, doi.org/10.9707/2307–0919.1120.

5. Mary Lutyens, *The Krishnamurti Reader* (New York: Penguin, 2002), 61.

6. Jiddu Krishnamurti, *On Fear* (New York: HarperCollins, 1995), 69.

7. Pema Chödrön, "The Fundamental Ambiguity of Being Human: How to Live Beautifully with Uncertainty and Change." *Tricycle*, Fall 2012, https://tricycle.org/magazine/fundamental-ambiguity-being-human/.

8. Sen Hounsai Genshitsu, "Foreword." *The Book of Tea: The Classic Work on the Japanese Tea Ceremony and the Value of Beauty* (Tokyo: Kodansha International, 1989), 19–20.

9. Shunryu Suzuki, *Zen Mind, Beginner's Mind* (New York: Weatherhill, 1995), 43.

10. Suzuki, *Zen Mind, Beginner's Mind*, 43.

11. François Cheng, *Five Meditations on Death: In Other Words...On Life* (Rochester, VT: Inner Traditions, 2013), 47.

12. Ronald Mellor, *The Historians of Ancient Rome: An Anthology of the Major Writings* (London: Routledge, 2012), 365.

13. Josho Brouwers, "The Death of Seneca." *Ancient World Magazine*. February 9, 2018, https://www.ancientworldmagazine.com/articles/death-seneca/.

14. Lucius Annaeus Seneca, *How to Die: An Ancient Guide to the End of Life* (Princeton, NJ: Princeton University Press, 2018), 6.

15. Seneca, *How to Die*, 9.

16. Seneca, *How to Die*, 11.

17. Seneca, *How to Die*, 22.

18. Viktor Frankl, *Man's Search for Meaning* (Boston, MA: Beacon, 1992), 9.

19. Frankl, *Man's Search for Meaning*, 75.

20. Frankl, *Man's Search for Meaning*, 117.

21. Frankl, *Man's Search for Meaning*, 117.

22. Iddo Landau, *The Oxford Handbook of Meaning in Life* (Oxford University Press, 2022), 219.

23. Frankl, *Man's Search for Meaning*, 9.

24. Frankl, *Man's Search for Meaning*, 113.

25. Sallie Tisdale, *Advice for Future Corpses (and Those Who Love Them): A Practical Perspective on Death and Dying* (New York: Touchstone, 2018), 1.

26. Tisdale, *Advice for Future Corpses*, 173.

27. Lisa O'Carroll, "Boy Dies After Allergic Reaction to Cheese 'Forced' on Him at School." *The Irish Times*, July 11, 2017, https://www.irishtimes.com/news/world/uk/boy-dies-after-allergic-reaction-to-cheese-forced-on-him-at-school-1.3151270.

28. Tisdale, *Advice for Future Corpses*, 5.

29. Suzuki, *Zen Mind, Beginner's Mind*, 93.

30. Damien Keown, "The Meaning of Nirvana in Buddhism Explained." *Tricycle Magazine*, https://tricycle.org/magazine/nirvana-2/.

31. The Dalai Lama and Thubten Chodron, *Buddhism: One Teacher, Many Traditions* (Somerville, ME: Wisdom, 2017), 120.

32. Dalai Lama, *Buddhism*, 136.

33. Dalai Lama, *Buddhism*, 141–142.

34. Dalai Lama, *Buddhism*, 138.

35. Dalai Lama, *Buddhism*, 147.

36. Suzuki, *Zen Mind, Beginner's Mind*, 14.

37. Harold Aspiz, *So Long! Walt Whitman's Poetry of Death* (Tuscaloosa: University of Alabama Press, 2004), 73.

38. David Erdman, *The Complete Poetry and Prose of William Blake* (Berkeley: University of California Press, 2008), 490.

39. John Martin Fischer and Benjamin Mitchell-Yellin, *Near-Death Experiences: Understanding Visions of the Afterlife* (Oxford: Oxford University Press, 2016), 61–62.

40. Bruce Greyson, "A Typology of Near-Death Experiences." *American Journal of Psychiatry* 142:8 (1985): 967–969.

41. Pim van Lommel, "Getting Comfortable with Near-Death Experiences: Dutch Prospective Research on Near-Death Experiences During Cardiac Arrest." *Missouri Medicine* 111.2 (2014): 126–131.

42. Pirn van Lommel, "Near-death Experience in Survivors of Cardiac Arrest: A Prospective Study in the Netherlands." The Lancet 358.9298 (2001): 2039–2045, DOI:10.1016/S0140–6736(01)07100–8

43. Bruce Greyson, "Getting Comfortable With Near Death Experiences: An Overview of Near-Death Experiences." *Missouri Medicine* 110.6 (2013): 475–481.

44. Raymond Moody, *Life After Life* (New York: HarperOne, 2015), 123.

45. Bruce Greyson, "Defining Near-Death Experiences." *Mortality* 4.1 (1999): 7–19.

46. Bruce Greyson, "Defining Near-Death Experiences." *Mortality* 4.1 (1999): 7–19.

47. Jeffrey Long, "Near-Death

Experiences: Evidence for Their Reality." *Missouri Medicine* 111.5 (2014): 372–380.

48. Peter Fenwick, "End of Life Experiences and Their Implications for Palliative Care." *International Journal of Environmental Studies* 64.3 (2007), 315–323.

49. Bruce Greyson, "Defining Near-Death Experiences." *Mortality* 4.1 (1999): 7–19.

50. Bruce Greyson, "Defining Near-Death Experiences." *Mortality* 4.1 (1999): 7–19.

51. Bruce Greyson, "Western Scientific Approaches to Near-Death Experiences." *Humanities* 4.4 (2015): 775–796, https://doi.org/10.3390/h4040775.

52. Lisa J. Miller, *The Oxford Handbook of Psychology and Spirituality* (Oxford: Oxford University Press, 2013), 520.

53. Bruce Greyson, "Biological Aspects of Near-Death Experiences." *Perspectives in Biology and Medicine* 42.1 (1998): 14–32.

54. Bruce Greyson, "Getting Comfortable With Near Death Experiences: An Overview of Near-Death Experiences." *Missouri Medicine* 110.6 (2013): 475–481.

55. Bruce Greyson, "Getting Comfortable With Near Death Experiences: An Overview of Near-Death Experiences." *Missouri Medicine* 110.6 (2013): 475–481.

56. Mark Fox, *Through the Valley of the Shadow of Death: Religion, Spirituality and the Near-Death Experience* (New York: Routledge, 2002), 1.

57. Fox, *Through the Valley of the Shadow of Death*, 1.

58. Fox, *Through the Valley of the Shadow of Death*, 2.

59. Fox, *Through the Valley of the Shadow of Death*, 57.

60. Fox, *Through the Valley of the Shadow of Death*, 59.

61. Fox, *Through the Valley of the Shadow of Death*, 45.

62. Mark Fox, *Religion, Spirituality and the Near-Death Experience* (London: Routledge, 2003), 82.

63. Judith Cressy, *The Near-Death Experience: Mysticism or Madness* (Hanover, MA: Christopher Publishing House, 1994), 65.

64. Cressy, *The Near-Death Experience*, 63.

65. Peter Fenwick and Elizabeth Fenwick, *The Art of Dying* (London: Continuum, 2008), 213.

66. Fenwick and Fenwick, *The Art of Dying*, 221.

67. Dalai Lama, *Advice on Dying: And Living a Better Life* (New York: Atria Books, 200), 240.

68. Dalai Lama, *Advice on Dying*, 88–89.

69. Thich Nhat Hanh, *No Death, No Fear: Comforting Wisdom for Life* (New York: Riverhead Books, 2002), 126.

70. Hanh, *No Death, No Fear*, 3.

71. Hanh, *No Death, No Fear*, 19.

72. Kahlil Gibran, *The Prophet* (New York: Knopf, 1923), 81.

73. David Erdman, *The Complete Poetry and Prose of William Blake* (Berkeley: University of California Press, 2008), 251.

74. Mandy Harvey, *Sensing the Rhythm: Finding My Voice in a World Without Sound* (New York: Howard Books, 2017), 150.

Works Cited

Achen, Paris. "Turkey: Hazelnut Capital of the World." *Capital Press*, September 3, 2019, https://www.capitalpress.com/ag_sectors/orchards_nuts_vines/-turkey-hazelnut-capital-of-the-world/-article_2b403308-ce5e-11e9-bff9-1b26383e83a6.html.

Addiss, Stephen. *The Art of Haiku: Its History Through Poems and Paintings by Japanese Masters* (Boulder, CO: Shambhala, 2012).

Adler, Robert. "The Clean Water Act: Has It Worked?" *Environmental Protection Agency Journal* 20.1–2 (1994).

American Academy of Allergy Asthma and Immunology. *Allergy Facts and Figures*, https://www.aafa.org/allergy-facts/.

Annunziato, Rachel, et al. "Longitudinal Evaluation of Food Allergy–Related Bullying." The *Journal of Allergy and Clinical Immunology* 2.5 (2014): 639–641, doi.org/10.1016/j.jaip.2014.05.001.

"Anxiety Disorders." National Institute of Mental Health, https://www.nimh.nih.gov/health/topics/anxiety-disorders.

"Aravax Takes a Step Closer to Developing a Peanut Allergy Vaccine." *Pharmaceutical Technology*, March 9, 2019, https://www.pharmaceutical-technology.com/comment/aravax-takes-a-step-closer-to-developing-a-peanut-allergy-vaccine/www.nimh.nih.gov/health/topics/anxiety-disorders.

Aspiz, Harold. *So Long! Walt Whitman's Poetry of Death* (Tuscaloosa: University of Alabama Press, 2004).

"Asthma." World Health Organization, https://www.who.int/news-room/fact-sheets/detail/asthma.

Ayshford, Emily. "Exploring Food Allergy Origins and Treatments." *Breakthroughs: Feinberg School of Medicine Research Office*, April 2019. https://www.feinberg.northwestern.edu/research/docs/newsletters/2019/april20191.pdf.

Banerji, Aleena, et al. "Predictors of Hospital Admission for Food-Related Allergic Reactions That Present to the Emergency Department." *Annals of Allergy, Asthma & Immunology* 106.1 (2011): 42–48.

Bartnikas, Lisa M., et al. "Impact of School Peanut-Free Policies on Epinephrine Administration." *Journal of Allergy and Clinical Immunology* 140.2 (2017): 465–473. doi: 10.1016/j.jaci.2017.01.040.

Bartuzi, Zbigniew, et al. "The Diagnosis and Management of Food Allergies." *Advances in Dermatology and Allergology* 34.5 (2017): 391–404. doi: 10.5114/ada.2017.71104.

Bennett, Patrick. "Developing an Adult Food Allergy Is a Life-Changer." *Allergic Living*, https://www.allergicliving.com/2016/01/19/when-allergy-strikes-an-adult/.

Bray, Bethany. "Supporting Clients Through the Anxiety and Exhaustion of Food Allergies." *Counseling Today*, November 27, 2018, https://ct.counseling.org/category/counseling-today/.

Brouwers, Josho "The Death of Seneca." *Ancient World Magazine*, February 9, 2018, https://www.ancientworldmagazine.com/articles/death-seneca/.

Campbell, Benjamin. *Richmond's*

Works Cited

Unhealed History (Richmond, VA: Brandylane Publishers, 2012).

Chad, Zave. "Allergies in Children." *Paediatrics & Child Health* 6.8 (2001): 555–566. doi: 10.1093/pch/6.8.555.

Chambers, John Whiteclay. *The Oxford Companion to American Military History* (Oxford University Press, 2000).

Cheng, François. *Five Meditations on Death: In Other Words...On Life* (Rochester, VT: Inner Traditions, 2013).

Chödrön, Pema. "The Fundamental Ambiguity of Being Human: How to Live Beautifully with Uncertainty and Change." *Tricycle*, Fall 2012, https://tricycle.org/magazine/fundamental-ambiguity-being-human/.

Chung, Man Cheung, et al. "Trauma Exposure Characteristics, Past Traumatic Life Events, Coping Strategies, Posttraumatic Stress Disorder, and Psychiatric Comorbidity Among People with Anaphylactic Shock Experience." *Comprehensive Psychiatry* 52.4 (2011): 394–404.

Cianferoni, Antonella, and Antonella Muraro. "Food-Induced Anaphylaxis." *Immunology and Allergy Clinics of North America* 32.1 (2012): 165–195. doi: 10.1016/j.iac.2011.10.002.

Clark, Sunday, et al. "Frequency of US Emergency Department Visits for Food-related Acute Allergic Reactions." *The Journal of Allergy and Clinical Immunology* 127.3 (2011): 682–683. doi: 10.1016/j.jaci.2010.10.040.

Cleveland Clinic. "How to Help Your Child Deal with Food Allergy Bullying." November 5, 2020, https://health.clevelandclinic.org/is-your-child-being-bullied-because-of-food-allergies-5-tips/.

Clowes, Gina. "Siblings and Food Allergies: Don't Overlook Needs of Your Non-Allergic Child." *Allergic Living*, September 9, 2018, https://www.allergicliving.com/2018/09/19/siblings-and-food-allergies-dont-overlook-the-needs-of-your-non-allergic-child/.

Collins, Lisa Cipriano. *Caring for Your Child with Severe Food Allergies* (New York: Wiley, 1999).

Connell, Caroline. "Food Allergy Bullying at School Is on the Rise." *Allergic Living*, September 17, 2012, https://www.allergicliving.com/2012/09/17/food-allergy-bullying-on-the-rise/.

Cooper, Rose A., Elizabeth A. Kensinger, and Maureen Ritchey. "Memories Fade: The Relationship Between Memory Vividness and Remembered Visual Salience." *Psychological Science* 30.5 (2019): 657–668.

Cressy, Judith. *The Near-Death Experience: Mysticism or Madness* (Hanover, MA: Christopher Publishing House, 1994).

Crowther, Gillian. *Eating Culture: An Anthropological Guide to Food* (University of Toronto Press, 2013).

Cummings, A.J. "The Psychosocial Impact of Food Allergy and Food Hypersensitivity in Children, Adolescents and Their Families: A Review." *Allergy: The European Journal of Allergy and Critical Immunology* 65 (2010): 933–945, doi.org/10.1111/j.1398–9995.2010.02342.x.

Dalai Lama. *Advice on Dying: And Living a Better Life* (New York: Atria Books, 2000).

Dalai Lama, and Thubten Chodron. *Buddhism: One Teacher, Many Traditions* (Somerville, ME: Wisdom, 2017).

Danovich, Tove. "Parents, Schools Step Up Efforts to Combat Food-Allergy Bullying." *National Public Radio*, June 5, 2018, https://www.npr.org/sections/thesalt/2018/06/05/613933607/-parents-schools-step-up-efforts-to-combat-food-allergy-bullying.

Davies, Barbara. "I Can't Forgive the Cruel Bully Who Killed My Son." *Daily Mail*, May 10, 2019, https://www.dailymail.co.uk/news/article-7016559/-Mother-boy-13-died-pupil-threw-cheese-says-forgive-bully.html.

Dean, Jennifer, et al. "Disclosing Food Allergy Status in Schools: Health-Related Stigma Among School Children in Ontario." *Health and Social Care in the Community* 24.5 (2016): e43-e52. doi.org/10.1111/hsc.12244.

Debras, Charlotte, et al. "Artificial Sweeteners and Cancer Risk: Results from the NutriNet-Santé Population-Based Cohort Study" *PLOS Medicine* 9.3 (2022): doi.org/10.1371/journal.pmed.1003950.

Eckhardt, Robyn. *Istanbul and Beyond: Exploring the Diverse Cuisines of Turkey* (New York: Houghton Mifflin Harcourt, 2017).

Eltagouri, Marwa. "Three Teens Charged with Knowingly Exposing Allergic Classmate to Pineapple." *Washington Post*, January 27, 2018, https://www.washingtonpost.com/news/education/wp/2018/01/26/3-teens-charged-with-knowingly-exposing-allergic-classmate-to-pineapple-she-was-hospitalized/.

Erdman, David. *The Complete Poetry and Prose of William Blake* (Berkeley: University of California Press, 2008).

Evra, Jennifer Van. "When Allergies Lead to Fear of Food." *Allergic Living*, July 2, 2010, https://www.allergicliving.com/2010/07/02/food-allergy-fear-of-food/.

Fenwick, Peter. "End of Life Experiences and Their Implications for Palliative Care." *International Journal of Environmental Studies* 64.3 (2007), 315–323.

Fenwick, Peter, and Elizabeth Fenwick. *The Art of Dying* (London: Continuum, 2008).

Feuille, Elizabeth, and Anna Nowak-Wegrzyn. "Allergen-Specific Immunotherapies for Food Allergy." *Allergy, Asthma & Immunology Research* 10.3 (2018): 189–206, doi: 10.4168/aair.2018.10.3.189.

Fischer, John Martin, and Benjamin Mitchell-Yellin. *Near-Death Experiences: Understanding Visions of the Afterlife* (Oxford University Press, 2016).

Fleischer, David M., et al. "Effect of Epicutaneous Immunotherapy Vs Placebo on Reaction to Peanut Protein Ingestion Among Children with Peanut Allergy." *Journal of the American Medical Association* 321.10 (2019): 946–955, doi: 10.1001/jama.2019.1113.

"Food Allergies." *CDC Healthy Schools*, https://www.cdc.gov/healthyschools/foodallergies/index.htm.

"Food Allergies." United States Food and Drug Administration, https://www.fda.gov/food/food-labeling-nutrition/-food-allergies.

"The Food Allergy Epidemic." *FARE*, https://www.foodallergy.org/resources/facts-and-statistics.

"Food Problems: Is It an Allergy or Intolerance?" Cleveland Clinic, https://my.clevelandclinic.org/health/diseases/10009-food-problems-is-it-an-allergy-or-intolerance.

Fox, Jeremy K., and Carrie Masia Warner. "Food Allergy and Social Anxiety in a Community Sample of Adolescents." *Children's Health Care* 46.1 (2017): 93–107, http://dx.doi.org/10.1080/02739615.2015.1124773.

Fox, Mark. *Religion, Spirituality and the Near-Death Experience* (London: Routledge, 2003).

Fox, Mark. *Through the Valley of the Shadow of Death: Religion, Spirituality and the Near-Death Experience* (New York: Routledge, 2002).

Frankl, Viktor. *Man's Search for Meaning* (Boston: Beacon, 1992).

Frazier, Claude A. *Coping with Food Allergy* (New York: Quadrangle, 1985).

Friedlander, Adam. "2020: Undeclared Allergens Continue to Be the Leading Cause of U.S. Food Recalls." *The Food Industry Association*, November 19, 2020, https://www.fmi.org/blog/view/fmi-blog/2020/11/19/2020-undeclared-allergens-continue-to-be-the-leading-cause-of-u.s.-food-recalls.

Gagné, Claire. "Dr. Li and Her Chinese Herbal Remedies." *Allergic Living*, December 15, 2015, https://www.allergicliving.com/2015/12/15/dr-li-and-her-chinese-herbal-remedies/.

Gallagher, Michael, et al. "Strategies for Living with the Risk of Anaphylaxis in Adolescence: Qualitative Study of Young People and Their Parents." *Primary Care Respiratory Journal* 21.4 (2012): 392–397.

Galli, Stephen J., Mindy Tsai, and Adrian M. Piliponsky. "The Development of Allergic Inflammation." *Nature* 454.7203 (2008): 445–454. doi: 10.1038/nature07204.

Gao, Chungchan. *African Americans*

Works Cited

in the Reconstruction Era (New York: Routledge, 2016).

Genshitsu, Sen Hounsai. "Foreword." *The Book of Tea: The Classic Work on the Japanese Tea Ceremony and the Value of Beauty* (Tokyo: Kodansha International, 1989), 19–20.

Gibran, Kahlil. *The Prophet* (New York: Knopf, 1923).

Gire, James. "How Death Imitates Life: Cultural Influences on Conceptions of Death and Dying." *Online Readings in Psychology and Culture* 6.2 (2014): 1–22, doi.org/10.9707/2307–0919.1120.

Gray, Jeffrey Alan. *The Psychology of Fear and Stress* (Cambridge University Press, 1987), p. 208.

Greiwe, Justin. "Oral Food Challenges in Infants and Toddlers." in *Pediatric Allergy: Immunology and Allergy Clinics* (Philadelphia: Elsevier Health Sciences, 2019), p. 481–493.

Greyson, Bruce. "Biological Aspects of Near-Death Experiences." *Perspectives in Biology and Medicine* 42.1 (1998): 14–32.

Greyson, Bruce. "Defining Near-Death Experiences." *Mortality* 4.1 (1999): 7–19.

Greyson, Bruce. "Getting Comfortable with Near Death Experiences: An Overview of Near-Death Experiences." *Missouri Medicine* 110.6 (2013): 475–481.

Greyson, Bruce. "A Typology of Near-Death Experiences." *American Journal of Psychiatry* 142:8 (1985): 967–969.

Greyson, Bruce. "Western Scientific Approaches to Near-Death Experiences." *Humanities* 4.4 (2015): 775–796, doi.org/10.3390/h4040775.

Ham, Paul. *Hiroshima Nagasaki: The Real Story of the Atomic Bombings and Their Aftermath* (New York: St. Martin's, 2014).

Handwerk, Brian. "Why Do Humans Have Allergies? Parasite Infections May Be the Trigger." *Smithsonian Magazine*, October 29, 2015, https://www.smithsonianmag.com/science-nature/why-do-humans-have-allergies-parasite-infections-trigger-180957101/.

Hanh, Thich Nhat. *No Death, No Fear: Comforting Wisdom for Life* (New York: Riverhead Books, 2002).

Hannaway, Paul J. *Asthma—An Emerging Epidemic: A Manual for Patients with Asthma, Parents of Children with Asthma, Asthma Educators, Health-care Providers, School Nurses and Coaches* (Lighthouse Point, FL: Lighthouse Press, 2002).

Harvey, Mandy. *Sensing the Rhythm: Finding My Voice in a World Without Sound* (New York: Howard Books, 2017).

Hasler, Gregor, et al. "Asthma and Panic in Young Adults: A 20-Year Prospective Community Study." *American Journal of Respiratory and Critical Care Medicine* 171.11 (2005): 1224–1230. doi: 10.1164/rccm.200412–1669OC.

Hazlett-Stevens, Holly. *Psychological Approaches to Generalized Anxiety Disorder: A Clinician's Guide to Assessment and Treatment* (New York: Springer, 2008), p. 147.

Heller, Susie. "A Teen Died After Accidentally Eating a Chips Ahoy! Cookie Containing Peanuts." *Business Insider*, July 18, 2018, https://www.businessinsider.com/teen-died-after-eating-chips-ahoy-cookie-with-peanuts-2018-7.

Herbert, Linda J., and Lynnda M. Dahlquist. "Perceived History of Anaphylaxis and Parental Overprotection, Autonomy, Anxiety, and Depression in Food Allergic Young Adults." *Journal of Clinical Psychology in Medical Settings* 15 (2008): 261–269, doi.org/10.1007/s10880–008–9130-y.

Hockenbury, Don H., and Sandra E. Hockenbury. *Psychology* (New York: Worth Publishers, 2003).

Holland, Kimberly. "The Furor Over the Peter Rabbit 'Food Allergy Scene,'" *Healthline*, February 23, 2018.

Howard-Ruben, Josephine. "The Dangers of Flying While Allergic." *Scientific American*, February 13, 2019, https://blogs.scientificamerican.com/observations/the-dangers-of-flying-while-allergic/.

Howe, Lauren, et al. "Changing Patient Mindsets About Non–Life-Threatening Symptoms During Oral Immunotherapy: A Randomized Clinical Trial."

The Journal of Allergy and Clinical Immunology 7.5 (2019): 1550–1559, doi: 10.1016/j.jaip.2019.01.022.

Javanbakht, Arash, and Linda Saab. "What Happens in the Brain When We Feel Fear, and Why Some of Us Just Can't Get Enough of It." *Smithsonian Magazine*, October 27, 2017, https://www.smithsonianmag.com/science-nature/what-happens-brain-feel-fear-180966992/.

Kane, Jeremy C., et al. "A Scoping Review of Health-related Stigma Outcomes for High-burden Diseases in Low- and Middle-income Countries." *BMC Medicine* 17 (2019): 17. doi: 10.1186/s12916-019-1250-8.

Kemp, Stephen F., Richard F. Lockey, and Estelle R. Simons. "Epinephrine: The Drug of Choice for Anaphylaxis—A Statement of the World Allergy Organization." *The World Allergy Organization Journal* Volume 1, Supplement 2 (2008): S18-S26. doi.org/10.1186/1939–4551-1-S2-S18.

Keown, Damien. "The Meaning of Nirvana in Buddhism Explained." *Tricycle Magazine*, https://tricycle.org/magazine/nirvana-2/.

Kivi, Rose. "Acute Stress Disorder." *Healthline*, September 29, 2018, https://www.healthline.com/health/acute-stress-disorder.

Klass, Perri, "Life-Threatening Allergic Reactions Rising in Children." *New York Times*, April 9, 2018, https://www.nytimes.com/2018/04/09/well/family/life-threatening-allergic-reactions-rising-in-children.html.

Kondo, Naomi, et al. "Medical Treatment of Food Allergies Should Be Personalized." *Personalized Medicine Universe* 4 (2015): 73–75, doi.org/10.1016/j.pmu.2015.03.005.

Krishnamurti, Jiddu. *On Fear* (New York: HarperCollins, 1995).

Krishnamurti, Jiddu. "3rd Question & Answer Meeting." Switzerland—July 26, 1983, https://jkrishnamurti.org/content/3rd-question-answer-meeting-14.

Landau, Iddo. *The Oxford Handbook of Meaning in Life* (Oxford University Press, 2022).

Landhuis, Esther. "Could Your Mindset Affect How Well a Treatment Works?" *National Public Radio*, March 1, 2019, https://www.npr.org/sections/health-shots/2019/03/01/699399504/could-your-mindset-affect-how-well-a-treatment-works.

Lange, Lars. "Quality of Life in the Setting of Anaphylaxis and Food Allergy." *Allergo Journal International* 23.7 (2014): 252–260. doi: 10.1007/s40629–014–0029-x.

Lapinsky, Stephen E. "Endotracheal Intubation in the ICU." *Critical Care* 19.1 (2015): 258. doi: 10.1186/s13054–015–0964-z.

Larsen, Jørgen Nedergaard, et al. "Allergy Immunotherapy: The Future of Allergy Treatment." *Drug Discovery Today* 21.1 (2016): 26–37, doi.org/10.1016/j.drudis.2015.07.010.

Lee, Khui Hung, et al. "The Gut Microbiota, Environmental Factors, and Links to the Development of Food Allergy." *Clinical and Molecular Allergy* 18.5 (2020): 1–11, doi.org/10.1186/s12948–020–00120-x.

Lee, Youngsoo, et al. "A Prospective Observation of Psychological Distress in Patients with Anaphylaxis." *Allergy, Asthma & Immunology Research* 12.3 (2020): 496–506, doi: 10.4168/aair.2020.12.3.496.

Leo, Harvey L., and Noreen M. Clark. "Managing Children with Food Allergies in Childcare and School." *Current Allergy & Asthma Reports* 7 (2007): 187–191, doi: 10.1007/s11882–007–0020–4.

Lieberman, Jay A., et al. "Bullying Among Pediatric Patients with Food Allergy." Annals of *Allergy, Asthma & Immunology* 105.4 (2010): 282–286, doi.org/10.1016/j.anai.2010.07.011.

Lieberman, Jay A., et al. "The Global Burden of Illness of Peanut Allergy: A Comprehensive Literature Review." *Allergy: The European Journal of Allergy and Critical Immunology* 76 (2021): 1367–1384, doi.org/10.1111/all.14666.

Lieberman, Phil. "Reactions to Peanut During Air Travel: Can Anaphylaxis Be Due to Inhalation?"

Works Cited

American Academy of Allergy, Asthma & Immunology, https://www.aaaai.org/-allergist-resources/ask-the-expert/answers/old-ask-the-experts/peanut-air-travel.

Liem, Djin Gie, and Catherine Georgina Russell. "The Influence of Taste Liking on the Consumption of Nutrient Rich and Nutrient Poor Foods." *Frontiers in Nutrition,* November 15, 2019, doi.org/10.3389/fnut.2019.00174.

Lisann, Lauren, et al. "Successful Prevention of Extremely Frequent and Severe Food Anaphylaxis in Three Children by Combined Traditional Chinese Medicine Therapy." *Allergy, Asthma & Clinical Immunology* 10 (2014): 1–11, doi.org/10.1186/s13223–014–0066–5.

Lomas, Jeanne and Kirsi Järvinen. "Managing Nut-induced Anaphylaxis: Challenges and Solutions." *Journal of Asthma and Allergy* 8 (2015): 115–123, doi: 10.2147/JAA.S89121.

Lommel, Pim van. "Getting Comfortable with Near-Death Experiences: Dutch Prospective Research on Near-Death Experiences During Cardiac Arrest." *Missouri Medicine* 111.2 (2014): 126–131.

Lommel, Pirn van. "Near-death Experience in Survivors of Cardiac Arrest: A Prospective Study in the Netherlands." *The Lancet* 358.9298 (2001): 2039–2045, DOI:10.1016/S0140–6736(01)07100–8.

Long, Jeffrey. "Near-Death Experiences: Evidence for Their Reality." *Missouri Medicine* 111.5 (2014): 372–380.

Lopez, Mary Stachyra. *Images of America: Centreville and Chantilly* (Charlestown, SC: Arcadia, 2014).

Lutyens, Mary. *The Krishnamurti Reader* (New York: Penguin, 2002).

Masia, Carrie L. et al. "Peanut Allergy in Children: Psychological Issues and Clinical Considerations." *Education and Treatment of Children* 21.4 (1998): 514–531.

Matti, Mariam. "Michigan Student Pleads Guilty in Peanut Butter Face-Smearing Case." *Allergic Living,* September 6, 2017, https://www.allergicliving.com/2017/09/06/michigan-student-pleads-guilty-in-peanut-butter-face-smearing-case/.

Mehta, Harshna. "Growth and Nutritional Concerns in Children with Food Allergy." *Current Opinion in Allergy and Clinical Immunology* 13.3 (2013): 275–279, doi: 10.1097/ACI.0b013e328360949d.

Mellor, Ronald. *The Historians of Ancient Rome: An Anthology of the Major Writings* (London: Routledge, 2012).

Miller, Lisa J. *The Oxford Handbook of Psychology and Spirituality* (Oxford University Press, 2013).

Mitrea, Lilieana Stadler. *Pharmacology* (Ontario: Natural Medicine Books, 2008).

Mondello, Wendy. "Girl with Milk Allergy Dies of Severe Reaction Related to Desensitization." *Allergic Living,* December 20, 2021, https://www.allergicliving.com/2021/12/20/girl-with-milk-allergy-dies-of-severe-reaction-related-to-desensitization/.

Moody, Harry R. *Abundance of Life: Human Development Policies for an Aging Society* (New York: Columbia University Press, 1988).

Moody, Raymond. *Life After Life* (New York: HarperOne, 2015), p. 123.

Moote, William, and Harold Kim. "Allergen-specific Immunotherapy." *Allergy, Asthma & Clinical Immunology* 7 (2011): 1–7, doi: 10.1186/s13223–018–0282–5.

Mousallem, T., and A.W. Burks. "Immunology in the Clinic Review Series; Focus on Allergies: Immunotherapy for Food Allergy." *Clinical and Experimental Immunology* 167.1 (2012): 26–31, doi: 10.1111/j.1365–2249.2011.04499.x.

Muraro, Antonella, et al. "Comparison of Bullying of Food-allergic Versus Healthy School Children in Italy." *Annals of Allergy, Asthma & Immunology* 105.4 (2010): 282–286, doi.org/10.1016/j.anai.2010.07.011.

Navinés-Ferrer, Arnau, et al. "IgE-Related Chronic Diseases and Anti-IgE-Based Treatments." *Journal of Immunology Research* (2016): 1–12, doi: 10.1155/2016/8163803.

New York State Department of Health. "Making the Difference: Caring for Students with Life-Threatening Allergies." https://www.health.ny.gov/

professionals/protocols_and_guide lines/docs/caring_for_students_with_ life_threatening_allergies.pdf.

Newman, Kristina L. "Beliefs About Food Allergies in Adolescents Aged 11–19 Years: A Systematic Review." *Clinical & Translational Allergy* 12.4 (2022): e12142, doi: 10.1002/clt2.12142.

"1981: Sus-Phrine: The Greatest Asthma Medicine Ever." *Asthma History Blogspot* http://asthmahistory.blogspot.com/2017/03/1981-sus-phrin-greatest-asthma-medicine.html.

Nwaru, Bright, et al. "Idiopathic Anaphylaxis." *Current Treatment Options in Allergy* 4.3 (2017): 312–319, doi: 10.1007/s40521–017–0136–2.

O'Carroll, Lisa. "Boy Dies After Allergic Reaction to Cheese Allegedly Forced on Him." *The Guardian,* July 11, 2017, https://www.theguardian.com/uk-news/2017/jul/11/karanbir-cheema-dies-allergic-reaction-cheese-allegedly-forced-on-him.

O'Carroll, Lisa. "Boy Dies After Allergic Reaction to Cheese 'Forced' on Him at School." *The Irish Times,* July 11, 2017, https://www.irishtimes.com/news/world/uk/boy-dies-after-allergic-reaction-to-cheese-forced-on-him-at-school-1.3151270.

Paddock, Catharine. "Hookworms and Allergies—Doctor Infects Himself for Experiment." *Medical News Today,* April 18, 2012, https://www.medicalnewstoday.com/articles/244238#1.

Pai, Anushka, et al. "Posttraumatic Stress Disorder in the DSM-5: Controversy, Change, and Conceptual Considerations." *Behavioral Science* 7.1 (2017): 1–7, doi: 10.3390/bs7010007.

Phelan, Jo C., et al. "Stigma, Status, and Population Health." *Social Science and Medicine* 103 (2014): 15–23. doi: 10.1016/j.socscimed.2013.10.004.

Plamper, Jan, and Benjamin Lazier. *Fear: Across the Disciplines* (Pittsburg, PA: University of Pittsburg Press, 2012).

Poniewozik, James. "Anthony Bourdain: The Man Who Ate the World." *New York Times,* June 8, 2018, https://www.nytimes.com/2018/06/08/arts/television/bourdain-death.html.

"Prednisone." National Library of Medicine, Medline Plus, https://medlineplus.gov/druginfo/meds/a601102.html.

Prescott, Susan, and Katrina J. Allen. "Food Allergy: Riding the Second Wave of the Allergy Epidemic." *Pediatric Allergy and Immunology* 22.2 (2011): 155–160. doi.org/10.1111/j.1399–3038.2011.01145.x.

Rabin, Roni Caryn. "For Children with Peanut Allergies, F.D.A. Experts Recommend a New Treatment." *New York Times,* Sept. 13, 2019, https://www.nytimes.com/2019/09/13/health/-peanut-allergy-children.html.

Rabin, Roni Caryn. "In Allergy Bullying, Food Can Hurt." *New York Times,* February 15, 2018, https://www.nytimes.com/2018/02/15/well/family/in-allergy-bullying-food-can-hurt.html.

Reddy, Sreedhar, and M. Anitha. "Culture and Its Influence on Nutrition and Oral Health." *Biomedical & Pharmacology Journal* 8 (2015): 613–620, doi.org/10.13005/bpj/757.

Rich, Adrienne. *Diving Into the Wreck: Poems 1971–1972* (New York: Norton, 1973).

Sadreameli, S. Christy, Emily P. Brigham, and Ajanta Patel. "The Surprising Reintroduction of Primatene Mist in the United States." *Annals of the American Thoracic Society* 16.10 (2019): 1234–1236.

Salo, Jackie. "Mom's Heartbreaking Warning After Daughter with Allergies Dies from Eating a Cookie." *New York Post,* July 16, 2018, https://nypost.com/2018/07/16/moms-heartbreaking-warning-after-daughter-with-allergies-dies-from-eating-a-cookie/.

Sampson, Hugh A. "Food Allergy: Past, Present and Future." *Allergology International* 65.4 (2016): 363–369, doi.org/10.1016/j.alit.2016.08.006.

Sampson, Margaret A., et al. "Risk-taking and Coping Strategies of Adolescents and Young Adults with Food Allergy." *The Journal of Allergy and Clinical Immunology* 117.6 (2006): 1440–1445.

Schettler, Ted. "Toxic Threats to Neurologic Development of Children." *Environmental Health Perspectives* 109. 6 (2001): 813–816.

Works Cited

Selgrade, Mary Jane K., et al. "Induction of Asthma and the Environment: What We Know and Need to Know." *Environmental Health Perspectives* 114.4 (2006): 615–619. doi: 10.1289/ehp.8376.

"Senate Joint Resolution No. 24: Celebrating the Life of Paul Benjamin Ferrara." https://www.richmondsunlight.com/bill/2012/sj24/fulltext/.

Seneca, Lucius Annaeus. *How to Die: An Ancient Guide to the End of Life* (Princeton, NJ: Princeton University Press, 2018).

Shu, D'Andra Millsap. "Food Allergy Bullying as Disability Harassment: Holding Schools Accountable." *University of Colorado Law Review*, February 1, 2021, Https://lawreview.colorado.edu/printed/food-allergy-bullying-as-disability-harassment-holding-schools-accountable/

Sicherer, Scott H. *Food Allergies: A Complete Guide for Eating When Your Life Depends on It* (Baltimore: Johns Hopkins University Press, 2013).

Sicherer, Scott H., et al., "Management of Food Allergy in the School Setting." *Pediatrics* 126.6 (2010): 1232–1239, doi.org/10.1542/peds.2010–2575.

Sicherer, Scott H., et al. "The US Peanut and Tree Nut Allergy Registry: Characteristics of Reactions in Schools and Day Care." *The Journal of Pediatrics* 138.4 (2001): 560–565, doi: 10.1067/mpd.2001.111821.

Sifferlin, Alexandra. "Doctor Infects Himself with Hookworm for Health Experiment." *Time Magazine*, April 18, 2012, http://healthland.time.com/2012/04/18/doctor-infects-himself-with-parasites-for-health-experiment/.

Silverstein, Jason. "Panera Put Peanut Butter on Girl's Sandwich Despite Severe Allergy, Leading to Hospitalization, Lawsuit Says." *New York Daily News*, June 6, 2016, https://www.nydailynews.com/news/national/panera-put-peanut-butter-girl-sandwich-allergy-suit-article-1.2663106.

Smith, Gwen. "Sabrina's Law: The Girl and the Food Allergy Law." *Allergic Living*, July 2, 2010, https://www.allergicliving.com/2010/07/02/sabrinas-law-the-girl-and-the-allergy-law/.

Stjerna, Marie-Louise. "Food, Risk and Place: Agency and Negotiations of Young People with Food Allergy." *Sociology of Health & Illness* 37.2 (2015): 284–297, doi.org/10.1111/1467–9566.12215.

Suzuki, Shunryu. *Zen Mind, Beginner's Mind* (New York: Weatherhill, 1995).

Tanno, Luciana Kase, et al. "Asthma and Anaphylaxis." *Current Opinion in Allergy and Clinical Immunology* 19.5 (2019): 447–455. doi: 10.1097/ACI.0000000000000566.

Taylor, Jessica, and Chrystal Lewis. "Counseling Adults with Food Allergies After an Anaphylactic Reaction: An Application of Emotion-Focused Therapy." *Journal of Mental Health Counseling* 40.1 (2018): 14–25, doi.org/10.17744/mehc.40.1.02.

"Theophylline." National Library of Medicine, Medline Plus, https://medlineplus.gov/druginfo/meds/a681006.html.

"Think Positive for Better Health: Changing Negative Thought Patterns to Positive May Boost Physical and Mental Health as Well as Lifespan." *Mind, Mood & Memory* 7.7 (2011): 3.

Tisdale, Sallie. *Advice for Future Corpses (and Those Who Love Them): A Practical Perspective on Death and Dying* (New York: Touchstone, 2018).

Troster, Heinrich. "Disclose or Conceal? Strategies of Information Management in Persons with Epilepsy." *Epilepsia* 38.11 (1997): 1227–1237, doi.org/10.1111/j.1528–1157.1997.tb01221.x.

Tupper, Jennifer, and Shaun Visser. "Anaphylaxis: A Review and Update." *Canadian Family Physician* 56.10 (2010): 1009–1011.

Tzoumis, Kelly. *Toxic Chemicals in America: Controversies in Human and Environmental Health* (Santa Barbara, CA: ABC-CLIO, 2020).

U.S. Environmental Protection Agency. "Learn About Polychlorinated Biphenyls (PCBs)." https://www.epa.gov/pcbs/learn-about-polychlorinated-biphenyls-pcbs.

Works Cited

U.S. Food & Drug Administration. "FDA Approves First Drug for Treatment of Peanut Allergy for Children." https://www.fda.gov/news-events/-press-announcements/fda-approves-first-drug-treatment-peanut-allergy-children.

U.S. Food & Drug Administration. "Food Allergies." https://www.fda.gov/food/-food-labeling-nutrition/food-allergies.

Vargas, Perla A. "Developing a Food Allergy Curriculum for Parents." *Pediatric Allergy & Immunology* 22.6 (2011): 575–582, doi: 10.1111/j.1399–3038.2011.01152.x.

Vickery, Brian P. "Sustained Unresponsiveness to Peanut in Subjects Who Have Completed Peanut Oral Immunotherapy." *The Journal of Allergy and Clinical Immunology* 133.2 (2014): 468–75, doi: 10.1016/j.jaci.2013.11.007.

Vozzella, Laura, and Gregory S. Schneider. "Virginia General Assembly Approves Medicaid Expansion to 400,000 Low-income Residents." *Washington Post,* May 30, 2018, https://www.washingtonpost.com/local/-virginia-politics/virginia-senate-approves-medicaid-expansion-to-400000-low-income-residents/2018/05/30/5df5e304-640d-11e8-a768-ed043e33f1dc_story.html.

Wang, Julie, and Andrew Liu. "Food Allergies and Asthma." *Current Opinion in Allergy and Clinical Immunology* 11.3 (2011): 249–254.

Weissman, Susan. *Feeding Eden: The Trials and Triumphs of a Food Allergy Family* (New York: Sterling Publishing, 2012).

Winland-Brown, Jill E., and Brian Oscar Porter. "Respiratory Problems." in *Primary Care: Art and Science of Advanced Practice Nursing,* eds. Lynne Dunphy, Jill E. Winland-Brown, Brian Oscar Porter, Debera J. Thomas (Philadelphia: F.A. Davis Company, 2015).

Winter, Greg. "F.D.A. Survey Finds Faulty Listings of Possible Food Allergens." *New York Times,* April 3, 2001, https://www.nytimes.com/2001/04/03/business/fda-survey-finds-faulty-listings-of-possible-food-allergens.html.

Wong, G.W. "Comparative Study of Food Allergy in Rural and Urban Chinese School Children." *Journal of Allergy and Clinical Immunology* 123.2 (2009): p. S32.

Yu, Wong, et al. "Food Allergy: Immune Mechanisms, Diagnosis and Immunotherapy." *Nature Reviews Immunology* 16.12 (2016): 751–765, doi: 10.1038/nri.2016.111.

Zhovmer, Alexander S. "Novel and Emerging Therapies for Food Allergy." United States Food and Drug Administration, https://www.fda.gov/vaccines-blood-biologics/biologics-research-projects/novel-and-emerging-therapies-food-allergy.

Index

Index

Index